ON FRIDAYS WE FAST

How to Reach Your Ideal Weight

Mike Woosley, Ph.D., CPT

On Fridays We Fast

How to Reach Your Ideal Weight

2nd edition
© 2017, Mike Woosley, all rights reserved.

Graphic Design by Jason Haker

First Edition (December 2017)

ISBN-10: 1974680142

ISBN-13: 978-1974680146

Nonfiction > Health, Fitness, and Diet >
Diets and Weight Loss

Contents

Introduction

Our current first-world societies have created a river of food that flows continuously at us. We use food for recreation, for reward, to cure boredom, and far beyond its historical narrow biological purpose of sustenance. We are biologically wired to be addicted to food. That ensures we eat food when it is available. Unfortunately, it's always available. No wonder we're overweight. Around 70% of US adults are overweight or even obese.

On the other hand 30% of adults are not fat. There are many reasons not to be fat. Health and well-being. Your appearance. The expense of food and treatment of health problems. The potential cost of your diminished success and productivity.

Here's the good news: This companion will teach, inspire, and motivate you to reach your ideal weight. I will assure you that in doing this, you'll find that the value of food as something that is enjoyable and rewarding actually increases when food isn't used only to satisfy an addiction.

This book is for you if you are even a few pounds overweight. That means it's for almost three quarters of US adults. It doesn't matter if you need to lose 20 pounds or 200 pounds. Both challenges are hard. The tools discussed here will ensure you can solve the problem if you decide to do it. I will help you irrespective of how much weight you need to shed.

In this book, I'll teach you to determine, reach, and maintain your ideal weight. There are only a few weapons you need to have in your arsenal. I'll talk about hunger and fasting, their evolutionary role, and how they figure into the equation that will make you successful.

Terminology is important, so I want to square the terminology I will use in this book. Everyone who needs to lose weight is "overweight". People who are very much overweight are called "obese". I occasionally use the term "fat" to describe both. "Overweight" and "obese" are defined by the US Centers for Disease Control in terms of a BMI measurement that I'll put into context in Chapter 2 (those "stock" cutoffs provided by CDC may not be relevant for you).

Where you fall on a scale and whether you are "overweight" or "obese" is somewhat irrelevant. I've found that many people who think they need to lose 10 pounds actually need to lose 20 to 30 pounds or more. So you may have more of an "opportunity" than you realize. What is important is knowing how much you need to lose, and I'll show you how to calculate your ideal weight in Chapter 2.

This companion aims to make the challenge of reaching that ideal weight easier, not more daunting. It's important to set the right goal if you want to be successful. If you have allowed yourself to get fat, you might feel embarrassed. I want you to feel motivated to fix this problem without apology. This companion can help ensure your success. This book aims to give you the tools and mental framework for success – not a rigid prescription of steps to follow that are to complex too fit into a permanent lifestyle.

Being overweight or fat impacts negatively how those around you perceive you. It impacts how others view your effectiveness. Your closest family see through your faults. Others often judge you on your weight. That impacts your success in life. It's a threat to your health. It hurts your enjoyment of life, your optimism, and your productivity. Whether you need to lose 40 pounds or 100 pounds, you've taken a critical step by using this companion, because you've decided to fix your weight. This book will give you all the tools you need to reach your ideal weight.

Some of us are overweight and need to act but don't quite realize it. (If you know people like that, please give them this book when you are done.) In Chapter 1, I'll explain how those of us who are a slightly overweight may not realize how those last 15 pounds can be significantly harming your quality of life. Reaching your ideal weight is critically important to your health, well-being, and outlook. The last 15 pounds you need to lose are just as important as the first 50.

The good news is that you have every tool you need to reach your healthy weight within your grasp. This book will teach you how to reach that weight --- your "ideal weight". It's going to empower you to understand that you can decide what you weigh. This is in contrast to many cookbook weight management approaches that direct you to follow a series of complicated steps with the hope your weight is acceptable when it's all done.

Knowledge is a critical first step. Most of us don't know our ideal weight, much less what living at our healthy weight entails, so it's impossible for us to realize it. Knowledge, however, is not sufficient to bring you to your ideal weight. You will need two other things: focus and motivation that lead you to the correct action. This book will help you with that also.

Focus and motivation. "Shit it sounds like it might be difficult." It's not as hard as I am making it sound. Once you make the decision to reach your ideal weight and have the knowledge needed to do it, it is quite straightforward. Here's why: there isn't actually a need to be overly engrossed by the mix of foods you eat, to cook complicated meals at home, or carve out large amounts of time for exercise. The most important thing is that you decide to live at your ideal weight, and enter the mindset to reach and stay there, using the correct tools.

Not everyone who reads this book will succeed. Everyone who reads, understands, and acts on a decision he or she has made will succeed. The book does not make a guarantee. Only you can make a guarantee, and you should make that guarantee to yourself. You need to decide you want to reach your correct weight, be healthier, feel better, improve your quality of life, and live longer.

What I will promise you is that if you are able to read and understand this companion, you will know and understand what you need to do to reach your correct weight. I will strip away every other illusion that you have about what you need to do to reach your ideal weight.

If you are fat, if you need to lose 100 pounds or more, you're probably starting to assume you have more work to do than someone who needs to lose 20 pounds, or someone who is already at their ideal weight. That's not accurate. The work for all people is substantially the same: reaching and maintaining your ideal weight. Those activities aren't that different. If you are a very fat person, you'll merely have to wait longer to see yourself getting where you need to be.

If you are overweight or obese, you are probably starting to assume that life at healthy weight sucks. "Shit, I'm being asked to take on a lifestyle, and worse it's the lifestyle of one of those health nuts that I want to punch in the face every day." That's also not accurate. Living at your healthy weight is enjoyable. It's not difficult. In fact 68% of persons in the National Weight Control Registry (Chapter 8) who took off an average of 66 pounds and kept it off for over 5 years called maintaining their new weight "easy" or "moderately easy". If you've been weighing 300 pounds for 5 years (or 175 pounds), you've also been maintaining your weight successfully, even if it's not your ideal weight. Reaching and maintaining your ideal weight is not fueled by an addiction to excessive exercise. And it is full of rewarding food and the stuff that you liked to eat while you were fat. In fact, as you will learn, food actually becomes more rewarding when you live at your ideal weight. That's because we are all addicted to food, and people who eat (smoke, drink, take drugs) addictively never enjoy the activity as much as people who ration such rewards.

I am not recommending with this companion the necessity of any programs, systems, software, diet plan, supplements, meals, meal programs, meal replacements, paid exercise plans or any of the other paraphernalia of the diet industry. Some of this stuff is great by the way. It's just that its ancillary stuff that keeps you sane. It doesn't get you to your ideal weight. Only you do that. Many people who have been fat for years do Weight Watchers and drink Slim Fast, and many healthy people don't need these things. The inverses are also true.

My goal with this companion is to make sure you have the following tools:

- *An ability to calculate your ideal weight,*
- *An understanding what you have to do to reach your ideal weight,*
- *A comprehensive sense of how your action drives the outcome,*
- *The tools, motivation, and focus for success without distraction.*

I take this point further to say that while I recognize, you may decide that you want to use some of the tools, devices, and gimmicks of the diet industry because you enjoy them, or because they help you get through your day, or because they motivate you, that's just a personal choice. That's ok. Some days, a cup of coffee helps me get through my day. But you will do it without any illusions or distractions that you need this assistance to reach and maintain your ideal weight, and with the joy and empowerment of knowing that you have succeeded on your own terms, by your own force of will, and within your own control. (About half the successful folks in the National Weight Control Registry *who were successful for over 5 years didn't use any gimmicks at all.)*

How This Book is Organized. *The first chapter of "On Fridays We Fast" is just here to tell you why you should reach your ideal weight. Some of this material is already familiar to you, plus if you are reading already, you may have already decided to reduce your weight. That being said, I recommend you read it. It puts a little more specific dimension on the health issues, and will illuminate impacts your weight has on your health that you might not realize. It also addresses some of the social and success impacts of weight control that – because they are "non-PC" most resources on weight management omit these reminders.*

This book is presented as a handbook. Each chapter ends with quick exercises or thought provokers that will help you cement your commitment to reach your ideal weight. The great thing about the book is that each chapter gets more interesting than the previous chapter. The book starts out kind of boring, but by the time you get to Chapter 4 or 5, you won't want to put it down.

Chapter 2 and Chapter 3 are the companion chapters. These chapters will teach you how to calculate your ideal weight, and roughly how much food you can eat to maintain that weight. Important stuff to know. How could you succeed without a goal and measurement? Chapter 2 gives you a lot of background on BMI, why it is so useful, and how it needs to be customized to give a correct weight for men and women of differing body compositions. It's ok to skim it if you want, but make sure you finish it with a calculation of your own ideal weight which comes from Table 5. Chapter 3 enables you to calculate roughly how much food you can eat every day (in total calories) to reach your ideal weight at a steady pace. Counting the calories of everything you eat is very difficult, and knowing if you've calculated the correct allowable calories for yourself is also uncertain: it requires knowing something called your Resting Metabolic Rate which can only be easily estimated. An error of 500 calories per day is extremely significant. So this guide gives you a target level of calories, which you will tweak via experience.

Chapters Chapter 4 and Chapter 5 give you the first two arrows in your quiver of success: how to use hunger and fasting to reach your goals.

Chapter 6 talks about nutrition. While there is a lot of great information on eating and health, it's ok to skim this one as well and just read the summary at the end. This would not be a companion if it weren't ok to skip around. One of the key messages of Chapter 6 is that if you are not at your ideal weight, it's a waste of time to place obsessive focus on what you eat, when the only thing that impacts your weight is how much you eat.

Chapter 7 talks about exercise – one of the last arrows in your quiver. The information in the chapter discusses the role of exercise in reaching your ideal weight. Success is not possible if you don't understand the role of exercise. The good news, if you hate to exercise, is that you don't have to exercise very much to reach an ideal weight.

Many programs and systems to help you lose wait fail because they are too complex and too prescriptive, especially around food and exercise. On Fridays We Fast … recognizes that we are all individuals. This companion provides the tools necessary to succeed that work for everyone, recognize that people are different, and enable you to succeed with your own decisions and resourcefulness.

Chapter 1 – Why to Reach Your Ideal Weight

I debated whether I should include a chapter in this guide on why you should stop being overweight, because I am sensitive about wasting any person's time ... especially if you need to get focused on actually losing weight. If you're here, you've already identified a need to lose weight. You may need help, and you want to know how to be successful.

That being said, I am going to give you a succinct and organized look at this important information, because I need you to keep it in sight: It will support your motivation, and more importantly I'm going to remind you some basic "politically incorrect" facts that mainstream resources on weight often omit.

Most reasons for losing weight can be boiled into three categories:

- YOUR HEALTH AND QUANTITY OF LIFE,
- YOUR QUALITY AND ENJOYMENT OF LIFE, and
- YOUR SUCCESS IN LIFE.

Clearly, these categories aren't at all independent. If you are healthy, you have a better quality of life. If you are successful, you also have a better quality of life; however, there are worthwhile distinctions among the three legs of this virtuous stool.

Your HEALTH in this book more generally refers to objective measures of your physical condition: do you have diabetes? Is your heart healthy? What is your life expectancy (quantity of life)? Your QUALITY AND ENJOYMENT of life refers more directly to how you feel: do you have energy? Do you feel depressed? How is your libido? What is your level of desire to attack physical and mental challenges? Finally, your SUCCESS is linked to the outcomes that you achieve. You'll achieve better outcomes in most of your endeavors if you are at an ideal weight.

YOUR HEALTH AND QUANTITY OF LIFE

So many people are overweight or obese that we often see the statistics characterized as shocking. In the US, while statistics can vary from year-to-year, more than 35% of people are what the US Centers for Disease Control ("CDC") calls obese. Obesity is defined in the next chapter, but if you are more than 30 pounds overweight, you may be obese. (The CDC is a US federal agency charged with protecting American from health threats.) More than 70% of people are overweight or obese. Seven or more out of every ten Americans need to be read this book and act on what they learn. (If you are a European reader, these statistics are only somewhat better but they are trending worse on the continent as well.)

Here are diseases that research has shown are caused or aggravated by excess weight – and some of the impacts of having them. This list is not comprehensive.

CORONARY HEART DISEASE – you will need to spend most of your time sitting, because you can't exercise or walk up stairs. Your heart won't work well while you live, and then you will die an early death by gradually drowning due to poor pulmonary function;

DIABETES – obesity has a role in almost all Type 2 diabetes – and nearly 10% of US population develops it. When you get it, you'll have to constantly monitor and medicate your blood sugar... as you age, your extremities will lose circulation, and you'll face amputations and blindness.

CANCERS – breast, colon, others, are the worst way to die young

HYPERTENSION – high blood pressure, untreated causes organ destruction and death, pharmaceutical treatment can cause weight gain, impotence, and other fun side effects

STROKE – a bad guy! If you survive a bad one you might have to live permanently disabled, unable to walk or speak … you may even be a vegetable …until you are blessed by mortality.

LIVER AND GALLBLADDER DISEASE – these conditions can be chronic and deadly...likely caused by enzyme imbalances created in your body's management of a huge reserve of fat

SLEEP APNEA and breathing problems – lead to chronic feelings of exhaustion because you never achieve REM (deep) sleep, poor concentration, poor quality of life, constant sleepiness

OSTEOARTHRITIS – is an extremely painful disease that will cause your joints to deteriorate to bone-on-bone – and make even the most basic movement

excruciating …in the fat, this can be caused by your joints bearing undue
weight, or autoimmune problems, or both

GYNECOLOGICAL PROBLEMS (women) – abnormal periods and infertility are
caused by excessive body fat in women

ANDROGENIZATION (men) – low testosterone and libido, development of
feminine features and characteristics

DEPRESSION – chemical drivers of happiness and positive outlook are sapped in
the overweight

It's easy to look at this list and say – "Well shit, this looks like a list of all the things that might kill me. One of these will get me one day anyway." If you are still rationalizing like this now, you have no business continuing to read this book. It is acknowledged that not all fat people will suffer from all these ailments, but consider the following facts …

Some of these diseases are *stochastic* – for example cancer – you will either get it or you will dodge that bullet. So with those diseases, being overweight is simply adding more bullets to empty chambers in a game of Russian Roulette. If you do get cancer, you'll wonder if you would have developed it at your ideal weight. You have to decide whether you want to take these significant risks, or would rather like to live at your ideal weight.

Other of these diseases are *progressive*, which means you will be impacted by them to varying degrees no matter how heavy you are, if you are above an ideal weight. The fatter you are, the more impact you will see. One example might be arthritis. Even if you don't have a genetic predisposition for arthritis, if you are very heavy, the excess weight will wear the cartilage off your knee joints which simply are not designed for that load. When you are walking bone-on-bone, it is excruciatingly painful.

Most progressive impactors of being fat impact your QUALITY AND ENJOYMENT OF LIFE at some level depending on your level of obesity (**Table 1**). Someone 30 pounds overweight won't be able to keep up with their kids on a hike after those kids are about 10 years old. At 80 pounds overweight, you won't even be able to go on the hike.

DISEASE   NATURE

DISEASE	NATURE
Coronary Heart Disease	Progressive *(worse the fatter you are)*
Hypertension	Progressive
Liver and Gallbladder Disease	Progressive
Depression	Progressive
Sleep Apnea	Progressive / Stochastic
Osteoarthritis	Progressive / Stochastic
Gynecological Problems	Progressive / Stochastic
Androgenization	Progressive / Stochastic
Diabetes	Stochastic *(you get it or don't)*
Stroke	Stochastic
Cancers	Stochastic

Table 1 – Progressive / Stochastic Nature of Overweight-caused Illnesses.

A few of these ailments have both a stochastic element and a progressive element. Sleep apnea is a good example. Some people do not have a genetic predisposition for it; however if you do have a predisposition for it, the fatter you are, the worse it gets.

YOUR QUALITY AND ENJOYMENT OF LIFE

If you have heart disease, or a life-threatening cancer, it becomes quickly very obvious how your weight is impacting your health, quantity of life, and also quality of life. You feel worse and worse as your illness becomes more and more acute, you can't do the activities you enjoy, and your life expectancy is usually a few cancer-ridden years or less.

Even without an acute illness, if you are very fat – say you need to lose 100 pounds or more – you may manifestly realize that your weight is impacting the quality of your life. You feel uncomfortable in certain social situations. Air travel is either ideally avoided or impossible. You can't do well the functional things you need to live and care for yourself. You might need a wheelchair or scooter to make it through a shopping trip. Others perceive you as lazy.

But suppose you are just moderately overweight – 15 or 30 pounds. Your weight is impacting your quality of life and you may not know it. I've found this in scores of subjects I've interviewed. Sure "I don't feel good." "I can't play the sports and games I used to enjoy with my family." "I don't take hikes anymore." "I feel exhausted." But the rationalization is usually "My jobs too stressful", or "I'm getting older and these are just consequences of my age". A truly healthy person should not notice significant physical limitations of age until well into his 50's – but we're hearing these types of complaints for people in their mid-30's or younger.

If you are in this category, unfortunately your weight is subtly ruining your life. You are being brought down like the proverbial frog placed in the cold water before slowly boiling it: gradually but certainly.

US Marines, some of the best conditioned and most fit soldiers in the world are expected to carry a pack of around 50 pounds for an 8-hour march. If you are 30 pounds overweight, you are carrying most of the excess weight expected of a marine in battle --- except on a march that endures 24 hours per day, 7 days a week, 365 days per year while walking, sitting, eating, sleeping. No wonder you don't move much. No wonder you're tired. It's so basic and evident. Yet some people say, "It's because I'm getting older". No, it's because you got fatter.

If you are in this limbo of 30 to 50 pounds overweight, in some ways, you are in the worst place, because at least the truly fat know the cause of their horrible state of affairs.

If you're a man you are in a spiral of mediocrity. You don't feel as aggressive. You might not enjoy sports or physical activity as much – hiking, running, climbing – whatever you might ordinarily have enjoyed. If you are a woman, you may feel depressed or sad. You also won't feel energy and may feel disconnected.

Man or woman, you will see people around you at work, and wonder how they might have so much energy, curiosity and enthusiasm for what they are doing. You wonder how you can live up to the standards of others. It may even make you angry to see such enthusiasm around you. For yourself, you just want to get home and get on the couch so you can attempt to re-charge and start over the next day.

How did you get here? Again: like the frog in the boiling water. Maybe you had a sports injury or a minor surgery. You took your time to recover, gaining a few pounds. Maybe you had a lifestyle change: you got married, moved, started a new job, or had your first child and rationalized you no longer had time to exercise. I very often hear children used as an excuse: "We had kids and I no longer had time to exercise or focus on my health".

Here are the symptoms of what you have done to your quality and enjoyment of life with those first 30 pounds:

<u>In Nearly Everyone</u>

- Feeling tired and fatigued, carrying the marine pack
- Feeling alienated, sad, or mildly depressed
- Feeling lazy, tired, going to bed early
- Loss of libido and sexual energy

<u>Especially in Men</u>

- Lack of healthy feelings of aggressiveness – the type that make you want to compete, make you want to play sports, be successful at work
- Lacking the energy for day-to-day personal accomplishments and successes
- Feeling loss of self-confidence and force of personality

<u>Especially in Women</u>

- Clinical depression
- Anxiety and general continuous sense of frustration or powerlessness
- Loss of libido

If you've read this far and you can relate to any of this, you should be starting to feel motivated to improve your life. In Chapter 8, I am going to talk about motivation and focus to ensure you will succeed. It's appropriate to say that if you have used age, your job, your marriage, decisions about children, or any other lifestyle choice as an "explanation" (read that as "rationalization") for your excess weight, it's important that you let go of that false crutch. Your excess weight is only caused by what you stuff into your face.

Every week in the lifestyle section of the *Wall Street Journal* you can read a profile of a CEO or senior vice president of a large corporation in a state of ridiculously good health, and a description of how these men and women maintain diet and consistent exercise. Reading these profiles is humbling for me personally. These are men and women that have 100 times the level of responsibility of most of us, and many more demands diluting their time and attention than 99% of the rest of the population. They have wives, children, brutal careers, and community and social commitments; but they have realized that maintaining health and weight is key to their effectiveness, success, and well-being, so they've visualized that success and achieved it. People who tell me there is an issue of time, job, kids, corporate travel, eating in restaurants etc. are very much quite frankly whiners. We'll talk about how you can include exercise without wasting time or significantly changing your lifestyle in Chapter 7.

YOUR SUCCESS IN LIFE

This topic is the one that diet books and talk shows often don't like to talk address: The impact that your weight has on your success in life. In the previous section, I discussed how your excess weight erodes your energy for work and career.

Your success in life is also decisively predicated on how others around you judge you and view your effectiveness and credibility. This is impacted by your weight and appearance. Your weight impacts your career or social acceptance, and your interpersonal or romantic relationships.

How much impact your weight has on your success depends on how fat you are. In the first section of this chapter, I discussed how certain health effects of obesity are either stochastic (you get them or you don't) or progressive (the fatter you are the worse they are). For social acceptance, your weight has a progressive impact on your potential for general success: the fatter you are the more your potential for achieving your life goals is harmed by the biases of the people around you.

Career and Social Acceptance

In our society it has become nearly universally unacceptable to discriminate against people based on their race, gender, physical disability, or sexual orientation. It's also not socially acceptable to openly discriminate against a person based on their weight. That's a big part of the reason that this type of discrimination is not often discussed. Unfortunately, a lack of addressing this topic doesn't change the reality of how common and ubiquitous this discrimination actually is.

It's not my aim to condemn discrimination based on weight. Not only does it occur, it often has a rational basis. We are stuck with our race. Our weight is something we can control. The purpose of this discussion is to assert that the way to correct the problem is to correct your weight, rather than to spend the same effort meandering into an argument that people should not be judged based on weight or appearance.

When a person is seen as overweight, the person is perceived as not being able to control his or her immediate environment and impulses. Healthy persons, on the other hand, are perceived as having better control and more potential to be effective, which is important in job evaluations. Fat people are perceived as less in command, less organized, less able to sustain the stress of a challenging job, less attractive, and less conscientious. Even though interpersonal interaction in the workplace is usually non-romantic, the lesser attractiveness of an overweight person impacts the desire of potential co-workers to collaborate, interact, and visualize the fat person as successful in outward-facing roles.

If you are seeking a job or particular personal opportunity (appointment to a particular board, committee, or community opportunity), your weight puts you at a distinct and tangible disadvantage. I found more studies than I could count researching the effect of obesity or attractiveness on career attainment, wages, or even getting selected for a job. These were thoroughly researched studies appearing in prestigious journals like the *National Bureau of Economic Research*, the *International Journal of Obesity*, the *Journal of Applied Psychology*, the *Journal of Occupational Psychology* and many others. Conclusions like this one, from a study appearing in the *National Bureau of Economic Research* were typical:

> ...we find that a one percent increase in a woman's body mass results in a .6 percentage point decrease in her family income and a .4 percentage point decrease in her occupational prestige measured 13 to 15 years later. Body mass is also associated with a reduction in a woman's likelihood of marriage, her spouse's occupational prestige, and her spouse's earnings (Dalton Conley, 2015).

Further, and now I'm extrapolating, since healthy persons are more successful in career pursuits, you are more likely to be screened for a job interview by a healthy person as such persons are more frequently in decision-making roles. Studies have shown these persons or more biased against the obese. There is more bad news if you're a young women. Many of the studies seem to conclude that discrimination is worse against women, and worse against younger ladies than more senior women.

Acknowledge-ably, some of us are more gifted in personal attractiveness than others right out of the gate; however, even among persons with equal genetic gifts, the heavier we are, the less attractive we are. With each pound, we are moving ourselves down the success ladder.

If you are already in a job and getting fatter (hopefully if you've read this far, you are not actually blaming your job for your weight), you will find that you become less effective as you grow more fat. First, you have less energy. Next, people naturally do not want to work with people who are overweight, or otherwise appearing to lack control of their health. Co-workers don't want to go into battle with you, take those challenging business trips, meetings, or presentations with you as the key teammate. Over time, you'll find yourself not selected for the best career-moving challenges and the best opportunities, advancements, and promotions.

Again, I am not writing all of this to support or ratify discrimination based on weight or appearance, only to state that it is real, and the only way you can ensure you are not impacted by it is to operate at an ideal weight.

Interpersonal and Romantic Success

If you are seeking a mate, your weight is often a significant handicap. In the mating game, judgment based on appearance is less controversial than it is in the workplace. Men who are overweight are seen as less strong, effective, less in-control, and less capable to care for and protect a mate. Further, in men, excess weight is androgenizing. That means you look more feminine and actually have higher levels of female hormones and lower levels of male hormones. Women who are not at the correct weight are nearly always less attractive to men. Ideal weight in women sends signals to the man of youth, health, and fertility.

Sadly in the hunt for a mate there is often a mutual calibration. That means those who are overweight and seeking a mate may decide to settle for someone who is less attractive than their ideal, and also overweight. Not only do both persons have to compromise from a better ideal, but such unions often establish a cycle of obesity that passes to children.

Often just as dismaying are the cases where healthy young persons are married and then one spouse starts to become overweight. Typically the early relationship dynamic in weight gain is good natured-ribbing and trying to guide the fattening spouse from overeating. If your spouse is doing this to you, you should be assured that your weight has started to have an impact on your credibility, attractiveness, and sexual appeal to your mate. As this behavior evolves, the healthier spouse will often throw in the towel and start getting fat in a subconscious retaliation.

Over time there is not only a mutual loss of attractiveness and attraction, but also a mutual loss of respect that erodes the quality of the marriage. It's ironic that many divorcing couples lose weight and improve their appearance in conjunction with divorce, since focused and proactive behavior driven by shared mutual commitment to ideal weight could avert an erosion of marital attraction and affection in the first place.

Don't Let Your Weight Impede Your Potential

Notice that in the introduction to this discussion on how weight impacts success, I used the word "bias" not "prejudice" to describe how others perceive you. A bias, for or against perceived capabilities of a person, may be based on actual sound judgment that has – at least on a statistical basis – a legitimate foundation.

In other words, fixing your weight is not just a superficial objective to improve the way people perceive you, but actually a critical step you should take to improve your job abilities and effectiveness, and your inherent ability to attract, satisfy, and retain a mate.

Laslo Bock, who is the long-time head of HR at Google, is responsible for keeping over 50,000 employees at maximum productivity (and administers a program that provides free food and snacks to employees at work), had this to say in book *Work Rules!*:

> ANOTHER REASON I'M EMPHASIZING FOOD IS THAT DIET IS ONE OF THE BIGGEST CONTROLLABLE FACTORS THAT AFFECT HEALTH AND LONGEVITY IN THE UNITED STATES. MANAGING YOUR HEALTH, AND YOUR WEIGHT IN PARTICULAR, HAS ALL THE HALLMARKS OF AN IMPOSSIBLE TASK. ... IT REQUIRES SUSTAINED WILLPOWER ... AND WE'RE CONSTANTLY BOMBARDED BY SOCIAL PRESSURE AND MESSAGES THAT ENCOURAGE US TO CONSUME MORE.

While no person has control over his race or ethnicity, or an inherent physical disability, a person certainly has comprehensive control over his weight. (If you find yourself disagreeing with this statement, I promise your views will change after you read the next 7 Chapters.) It takes motivation and willpower. The same qualities that can make you successful at your job.

Why should you operate at any weight other than your ideal weight?

Exercises – Chapter 1 *Why to Reach Your Ideal Weight*

Completing these exercises will help you internalize activate the learnings of Chapter 1.

1. List five benefits you would expect to realize if you were at an ideal weight. You can list ideas discussed in Chapter 1, or you can think of your own.

1	
2	
3	
4	
5	

2. List two things you would like to do or have, that you can't easily realize due to your weight. If you are just a few pounds over your ideal weight, they don't have to be life changing, but they can be. If you are obese, they may be more transformational.

1	
2	

3. List or describe three ways you think your life would change positively for the better if you were healthier, more energetic, and living at your ideal weight.

1	
2	
3	

Chapter 2 – How to Calculate Your Ideal Weight

In this Chapter, I'm going to give you instructions on two methods to calculate your ideal weight. After you calculate your ideal weight you may be surprised at the resulting objective. Let me give you a bit of motivation: it's hard to be successful at anything if you don't set the right goal. I'm going to guide you to objectives that are aggressive and correct for you to maximize your health, quality of life, appearance and success. There isn't any reason to compromise for a weak goal or an intermediate goal.

As I've said earlier, controversy often arises in debate around the last twenty or thirty pounds. If you think you will be in good shape at 175, you may read the recommendations below and learn your ideal weight is 150 pounds. You may be skeptical. Let me make a couple of preemptive comments on why you should trust the recommendations here.

- First, don't assume that in the guidance provided, you are going for a scrawny runners build. This is not a book about calorie restriction. Muscularity is worthwhile for men and women. Good muscle volume improves functional strength, improves your metabolism, and – within reason – improves your attractiveness. The calculations and guidelines here incorporate your actual or desired muscularity. To be clear, the concept of ideal weight is a question of fat, not muscle.

- To further assert that the calculation of your ideal weight is not an aim to make you skeletal, note that in the most muscular athletes you see in *Sports Illustrated* or in the underwear ads of slick magazines, the reason you can see every abdominal, and every other muscle, is because these models are at an ideal weight without excess fat. Not because they have over-developed muscles. Attractive muscularity always involves a decision not to carry un-necessary fat.

- You may have a presumption based on the discussion so far that your ideal weight is hard to achieve. That's nonsense. The process for losing the last 30 pounds is the same as the process for losing the first 70, and the process for maintaining an ideal weight, and the amount of food eaten, is roughly the same whether you set that target weight at 150 pounds or 280 pounds. Once you reach any objective weight, the calories consumed to maintain it are the same. To be clear, you'd eat roughly the same daily calories to maintain a weight of 225 as you would to maintain a weight of 150 if your energy expenditure were constant (there is a difference in your resting metabolic rate when you are fat which we'll discuss in the next chapter). The daily calories actually may be more at 150 pounds than 225 pounds, since you'll have more energy and activity so that you will naturally burn more calories in your daily activities.

I'm going to provide you two simple mathematical method to calculate your ideal weight. The first method is anchored in the US Center for Disease Controls Body Mass Index ("BMI"). The second is based on your actual body fat. Both approaches are robust and will lead to similar calculations. The first one is easier to perform if you don't have access to an accurate means to measure your body fat.

BODY MASS INDEX

What the hell is BMI? The body mass index metric was first characterized by a Belgian engineer name Lambert Quetelet in the early 19th century (Devlin, 2009). It's a measure based on a ratio between your weight and your height. Quetelet originally proposed the metric to characterize the overall level of obesity of a population, rather than to characterize the individual. This is why, even though current BMI tables give ranges and not targets, BMI is often criticized as a tool not suitable for use in evaluating individuals. I'm about to tell you why it is a great tool for individuals.

Because BMI is quick and easy to calculate, and a meaningful tool in warning patients who may be overweight, the *National Institutes of Health* starting using BMI in the mid-80's. In 1998, NIH consolidated the guidelines, making the triggers the same for men and women, and the CDC officially adopted the metric. The biggest criticism of BMI is that because it does not take into account gender, or body composition (how much muscle you have), it may give false alerts for certain individuals. This discussion introduces modified-BMI to fix that problem. The second biggest criticism of BMI, is that it gives you a range of acceptable outcomes, so it is useless to tell you what you should actually weigh. I'm also going to fix that problem.

At this point, let's give a little bit of defense to BMI. Not only is it easy to use, but research has shown that it is a great predictor of body fat over large swaths of the population. For identifying the cut-off between "overweight", and "obese", I think that when it comes to the concerns about using BMI are a little academic: By the time you get close to the "obesity" cut-off you are very much overweight and are certainly going to have health impacts related to your weight. On the other hand, for the guidance on what is the beginning of "overweight", there is a difference between men and women, and muscularity also matters. That is why the guidance provided below is going to provide you with an ability to estimate a target BMI considering your gender and muscularity. In doing so, I supply a method to calculate your *ideal weight* instead of just your maximum allowable weight.

Understanding BMI

If you do use the BMI metric to evaluate an individual for weight, because BMI objectives are given in terms of ranges, you can only ultimately use the metric to determine your *maximum weight* … not your *ideal weight*. US CDC says that healthy weight is represented by a BMI of 18.5 to 25.0. That means if you have a BMI of 25.0, you are either healthy weight, or an ounce from being fat, depending on who you ask. Further, since the tool does not account for gender or body composition, if you are a woman, by the time you get to 25.0 you are probably already overweight.

In this section, I will better explain the genesis of BMI, explain why despite the fact it's often disparaged, that the metric is very useful, and I'll show you an easy way to calculate a modified-BMI that you can use to establish an ideal weight.

BMI is measured in kilograms per square meter (kg/m²). Here is the formula to calculate BMI:

$$BMI = \frac{Weight\ [in\ kilograms]}{(Height\ [in\ meters])^2} \qquad (Eqn.\ 1)$$

If you only know your height in inches and your weight in pounds, you can calculate your BMI this way:

$$BMI = \frac{Weight\ [in\ pounds]}{(Height\ [in\ inches])^2} \cdot 703 \qquad (Eqn.\ 2)$$

Here "703" is simply a single conversion factor that combines the conversion of pounds to kilograms and square inches to square meters into a single number.

The most common question about this metric is why in the hell do we divide our weight by the square of our height to calculate this metric? This measurement has been characterized this as completely arbitrary. A *National Public Radio* article called BMI "Scientifically Nonsensical" and went on to state "There is no physiological reason to square a person's height" (Devlin, 2009).

This accusation that BMI lacks a sound technical footing is not accurate, and squaring height does have a sound foundation in basic geometry. Think about the human body as kind of like a cylinder.

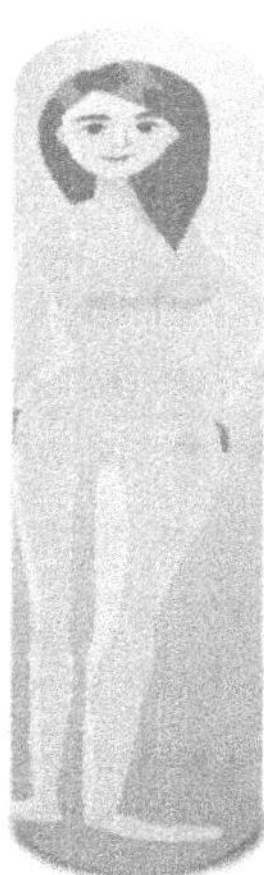

Figure 1 - *Human Body as a Cylinder*

Calculating BMI is kind of like un-rolling the cylinder of Figure 1 and using its surface area (**Figure 2**). If you remember your high school geometry, you remember that you can calculate the surface area of your cylinder like this

$$SA = \pi \cdot diamater \cdot height$$

Think of calculating BMI as dividing your weight by roughly your surface area to get your weight per unit of surface area. At this point you are going to say, "well in BMI we divide by *height* x *height,* not *π* x *diameter* x *height*".

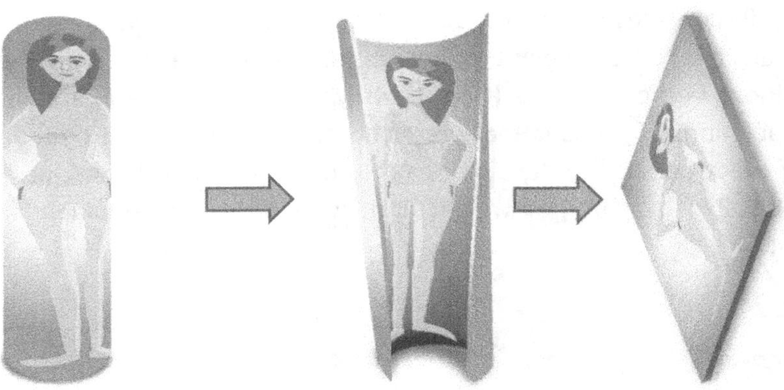

Figure 2 - *Calculating your "face weight".*

Here's why: when you look at the human body as a cylinder, your height is a good proxy for "circumference". For example, a six foot tall man has a diameter of about 2 feet. His "circumference" is *π•diameter = 3.14 x 2 feet ≈ 6 feet*, or approximately his height. This similarity is true over a wide range of heights. In general the taller you are, the greater your natural diameter.

If you ever buy carpet, you might know something about "face-weight" – which is the weight of the carpet per unit of area (grams per square foot, e.g.). Higher quality carpets have a higher face weight. Calculating your BMI is roughly calculating your face-weight, except that for carpet, more is better, and for people, more face-weight usually means overweight.

Why is the face-weight metric of BMI more useful than a simple un-squared ratio of weight to height? Using the height-squared metric allows us to quote suitable ranges of BMI that can be referenced by individuals, and that are independent of weight and height. For example, a BMI exceeding 25 (according to CDC) defines overweight for all people no matter your height. That would not be true if BMI were a simple ratio of weight to height.

Let me show you what I mean: Suppose we calculate a "linear-BMI" for individuals as simply defined as *weight / height*. In the two tables shown in **Table 2**, person who is 5'6" and 150 pounds has a traditional BMI of about 24. A person who is 6'2" and weighing 190 pounds also has a BMI of 24. Both are an acceptable weight according to the standard BMI ranges. On the other hand for linear-BMI the person who is 5'6 has a metric of 41, while the person who is 6'2" has a metric of 46. So using a plain [weight/height] BMI would require us to publish different objective ranges for every height of person.

The ranges of BMI suggested by the US *Centers for Disease Control*, allow us to compare the propensity of excess weight for persons of different heights using the same metric. The transitions in these metrics (from healthy to overweight, etc) are based on data for large populations of persons that are evaluated for the level of body fat, and the propensity of these persons to develop health problems related to weight. In this sense, BMI is a reliable indicator of weight and overweight for populations, while "linear-BMI" is not.

Actual BMI (height over weight-squared)

Weight in Pounds	height in inches				
	66	68	70	72	74
145	23	22	21	20	19
150	24	23	22	20	19
155	25	24	22	21	20
160	26	24	23	22	21
165	27	25	24	22	21
170	27	26	24	23	22
175	28	27	25	24	22
180	29	27	26	24	23
185	30	28	27	25	24
190	31	29	27	26	24
195	31	30	28	26	25

Linear BMI (height over weight)

Weight in Pounds	height in inches				
	66	68	70	72	74
145	39	38	37	36	35
150	41	39	38	37	36
155	42	41	40	38	37
160	43	42	41	40	39
165	45	43	42	41	40
170	46	45	43	42	41
175	47	46	45	43	42
180	49	47	46	45	43
185	50	49	47	46	45
190	51	50	48	47	46
195	53	51	50	48	47

Table 2 - Comparing BMI to "linear-BMI" - the real BMI is the same for every person of healthy weight, regardless of height – genius!

That being said, BMI is still an imperfect metric. I mentioned earlier that BMI was originally used to evaluate populations, not persons. This is why the ranges for acceptable BMI are very wide. For example, for a person who stands 5"7" tall, the range of acceptable weights ranges from 118 to nearly 160 --- that's a whopping 42 pound window.

Calculating your Ideal Weight using "Modified-BMI" method

So how the heck do I calculate my objective BMI? The BMI calculation is not sufficient to enable you calculate your ideal weight: (1) it omits key variables; and (2) it provides you only an objective range that is far too wide. We know that some people inside the acceptable range are fat. For a given height, persons at the low end of the range might be dangerously skinny, while persons on the high end of the range might actually benefit from losing substantial weight.

There are two metrics missing from CDC's generalized tables that, when considered, can enable you to use a BMI metric to narrow your ideal weight to within a few pounds: gender and muscularity. ***Gender*** is important because men and women have different natural body compositions. Healthy women carry more body fat than men – as much as 6% of body weight more. Healthy men naturally carry more muscle. Since muscle is 20% more dense than fat, men of a fixed height will have a higher healthy BMI than women.

The second factor to consider is ***Muscularity***. While men are as a general statement more muscular than women, there is a wide range of observed healthy muscularity in both men and women, and in fact, for men who are very muscular, their healthy BMI might even fall outside of the CDC range for healthy weight. For purposes of determining your ideal BMI and weight, it is necessary that you evaluate your own overall level of muscularity.

Muscularity is based on two factors: your natural body type, or "somatype" (from naturally skinny to naturally muscular) and how much you develop your muscularity through exercise or athletic activity. The combination of your natural body type, and how much you independently develop your muscle tissue determines your level of muscularity. For purposes of evaluating yourself, we are going to use six categories as shown in **Table 3**. These categories apply to men and women, and in reading the descriptions, you should be able to easily classify yourself in one of the categories with a bit of honest introspection.

Level 1	Level 2	Level 3	Level 4	Level 5	Level 6
Skinny / Runners' Build	Low Development	Average Muscularity	Athletic Build	Elite Athlete	Body Builder

Table 3 - Levels of Muscularity

These descriptions can help you verify your correct characterization in this continuum. Again, these descriptions are independent of gender and are generalized, recognizing that the amount of muscle on a female frame that belongs in the "body builder" category would be less than a man in the same category. Here is a little more description on the categories:

> **Skinny / Runner's Build** – if you belong in this category, you've probably been characterized as "skinny" or stick-like since you were a kid. You may exercise moderately or extensively, and you may have very good muscle tone,

but you just do not naturally carry a lot of muscle bulk no matter how much time you spend in the gym. Because people with this build are excellent runners and often self-select that sport, this build is often called a "runner's build".

Low Development – if you fall in this group, you may not have that "super skinny" or stick-like natural body of the runner. You are more likely to have an average body type, but you don't generally develop your muscles or keep them in tone via exercise or strength training. Whether or not you have a lot of fat on your frame, if that fat were stripped off, you would not see a lot of muscle mass on your frame and your muscles might be out of tone ("flabby" – don't worry, this is easily addressed in conjunction with weight loss).

Average Muscularity – if you belong in this category, you have either an average or perhaps low-athletic natural build or level of muscularity. Usually if you are in this group, you don't develop your muscularity specifically via strength training on a disciplined basis, but you have some strength or muscularity that is either natural, or the result of functional muscle development at work or via exercise (such as some level of recreational sports or activity).

Athletic Build – if you belong in this category, you may have an average build with plentiful strength training, or you have a naturally athletic build: you may be naturally muscular and you maintain your muscle tone via some level of recreational or competitive sports activity, and at least light to moderate strength training. A woman in this category may be engaged in cross-fit exercise that has significantly increased her natural muscular development.

Elite / Athlete – if you belong in this category, you are quite muscular or very muscular. You have at least an athletic natural build, and possibly a bulky / muscular build. Others would describe you as muscular. You may have engaged in very competitive athletic activity – such as college-level or very competitive sports. In addition, you've made an investment in strength training and probably spend time in the gym every week.

Body Builder – if you belong in this category, your natural body type is a very strong natural athletic build or more probably a stocky / muscular build. In addition, you spend substantial time strength training and you have substantially increased your muscle mass beyond natural levels by focused strength training. Whether you are male or female, the independent observer would characterize you based on your physique as a "body builder".

With this as background we have all the context and information we need to calculate a modified-BMI target and weight target based on your gender and muscularity. **Table 4** shows the old-fashioned ranges for BMI published by the CDC.

	BMI Range
Underweight	Below 18.5
Healthy Weight	18.5 to 24.9
Overweight	25.0 to 29.9
Obese	30.0 and Above

Table 4 - *Traditional CDC ranges for weight and obesity.*

Table 5 below is one of the most important figures in this book. It enables you to estimate a healthy body weight considering your height, gender, and muscularity. The old-fashioned method to evaluate your weight is to calculate your BMI based on your height and weight, and check to see if it falls inside the CDC healthy range. This tool takes as input not just your height, but also your gender and muscularity and lets you derive a targeted BMI and the corresponding healthy weight.

Here's an example from the table: if you are a man and you are 5 feet 9 inches tall, and your muscularity, based on the descriptions in **Table 3**, falls somewhere between a "3" and a "4", you should target an Ideal Weight between 149 and 156 pounds, or a BMI between 22 and 23.

Looking at the table, if you are a guy who is 5'9" and you characterize yourself as a "1" or a "2" in muscularity, you may look at the target weight of 135 pounds and react with surprise. If you're 40, you might say "I haven't weighed 130 pounds since I was in college." The same is true if you are a woman who is 5'7". You might also say "I haven't weighed less than 110 in years." Male or female, you've probably added a good amount of fat to your frame, and also lost some muscle mass.

There are a couple of important comments here. First, unless you are a serious runner who aims to maintain a seriously lean build, you really shouldn't be targeting "1" or "2" levels of muscularity. Greater muscularity improves metabolism, functional strength, and appearance. In this particular case study, for the male example, think of 130 as your foundational weight. It's the weight you would reach today at the correct body-fat percentage without addressing lack of muscle size and tone. **If you are extremely muscular – for men beyond a "6", you are off the right side of this table. There are a few of you out there. You need to use the body fat method in the next section to find your ideal weight.**

The philosophy for reaching your ideal weight, which you will read more about in Chapter 7, will be "fat first". Early exercise is intended to enable you to reduce fat. If you weigh 180 pounds and your ideal weight is 130 pounds, you should start shedding fat right away. It will eventually make sense for you to start improving your muscle mass and tone – not a difficult thing to do, and one we'll discuss more in Chapter 7 – but not worth a focused investment until you have lost 60- to 70% of the weight required to reach ideal weight.

male		muscularity					
	1	2	3	4	5	6	

female		muscularity				
	1	2	3	4	5	6

	BMI 17.0	BMI 18.0	BMI 19.0	BMI 20.0	BMI 21.0	BMI 22.0	BMI 24.0	BMI 28.0	BMI 30.0
4'10"	81	86	91	96	100	105	115	134	144
4'11"	84	89	94	99	104	109	119	139	149
5'00"	87	92	97	102	108	113	123	143	154
5'01"	90	95	101	106	111	116	127	148	159
5'02"	93	98	104	109	115	120	131	153	164
5'03"	96	102	107	113	119	124	135	158	169
5'04"	99	105	111	117	122	128	140	163	175
5'05"	102	108	114	120	126	132	144	168	180
5'06"	105	112	118	124	130	136	149	173	186
5'07"	109	115	121	128	134	140	153	179	192
5'08"	112	118	125	132	138	145	158	184	197
5'09"	115	122	129	135	142	149	163	190	203
5'10"	118	125	132	139	146	153	167	195	209
5'11"	122	129	136	143	151	158	172	201	215
6'00"	125	133	140	147	155	162	177	206	221
6'01"	129	136	144	152	159	167	182	212	227
6'02"	132	140	148	156	164	171	187	218	234
6'03"	136	144	152	160	168	176	192	224	240
6'04"	140	148	156	164	173	181	197	230	246
6'05"	143	152	160	169	177	186	202	236	253
6'06"	147	156	164	173	182	190	208	242	260
6'07"	151	160	169	178	186	195	213	249	266
6'08"	155	164	173	182	191	200	218	255	273
6'09"	159	168	177	187	196	205	224	261	280
6'10"	163	172	182	191	201	210	230	268	287
6'11"	167	176	186	196	206	216	235	274	294

Table 5 – "Modified-BMI": Ideal Weight and target BMI based not only on height, but also on gender and muscularity.

Trying to reduce fat and add muscle at the same time creates un-necessary work, creates confusion about whether your fat loss objectives are being achieved, and deprives you of the short-term motivation you get from seeing your weight decline as rapidly as possible. In the female example, if you are at a "1" in muscularity at 5'7", you should target getting below about 120 pounds before you address muscle tone, and then focus on replacing the last 10 pounds of fat with muscle so that your final target weight in the 120's.

BODY FAT MEASUREMENT – A GOLD STANDARD

I spent a lot of time talking about BMI and Ideal Weight for two reasons. Modified-BMI – a BMI target that also considers gender and muscularity is easy and accurate, and worthwhile in calculating an objective for ideal weight. You can calculate your modified-BMI target and ideal weight from the privacy of your own home without special tools and equipment.

To begin your journey to an ideal weight, it's a great way to get started, because it will give you very accurate objective weight. Maybe even the same weight you'd calculate with a body-fat measurement. As you get close to your ideal weight, especially if you are trying to improve muscularity as you shed final pounds of fat, having a good measure of body fat can be a huge help, and it can replace the BMI method of calculating an ideal weight with a more reliable measurement.

Unfortunately, all BMI-related measures are a proxy to measure how fat you are without actually calculating body fat. A body fat measurement is the gold standard for establishing a target weight. I will show you a way to calculate your ideal weight based on your objective level of body fat. I'm including this in the book because there are now cheap and highly available methods to actually calculate your body fat without using calipers (which are garbage). Once you know that ideal weight (by either modified-BMI or body fat measurement), you can target that weight with the correct dietary habits, and periodically check your body fat to confirm your results.

Calculating Ideal Weight using the "Body Fat" method

Let's get right into using your body fat to calculate your ideal weight. There are several methods to measure your body fat which I will address shortly. All methods calculate (or estimate) your body composition as two components: *fat* and *everything else*. "Everything else" includes skeletal muscle, bone, blood, organs and other fluids. Weight loss is focused only on fat. So say for example you weigh 200 pounds and have 30% body fat. You can theoretically never lose more than 60 pounds (30% of 200). Realistically you can never lose more than 45 pounds (because you can't survive without a certain safe level of body fat).

(There is a footnote on this two-component model of body composition which I will address at the end of this chapter and again in the chapter on nutrition. The upshot is this: depending on your size and existing diet, there may be an additional 10 pounds of variable weight other than fat relevant in understanding ideal weight. To give you a preview: people who eat a lot of carbohydrates tend to carry a lot of water weight, which is necessary to store the metabolic products of those carbohydrates. This variable weight is an overlay on the fat weight, which you need to permanently lose.)

In the modified-BMI calculation, you needed to consider your gender and your muscularity to determine an ideal weight and target BMI. With a body fat approach, you need only consider gender (because the body fat measurement measures your fat precisely without requiring your own self-assessment of your muscularity). Women naturally and necessarily carry more body fat than men, so the appropriate range of acceptable body fat is different for the genders. Women cannot menstruate or become pregnant without sufficient body fat, and sufficient fat creates curves on women that signal to men suitability for a mate. Men carry less body fat and naturally carry more muscle.

Table 6 shows you *typical* ranges of observed body fat for men and women. You can see from Table 6 that as people age, it has been observed that lean muscle declines and fat increases. Some would characterize this as a natural process, but a key driver of the process is that as we age, we become more sedentary. So it's actually a statistical association: old people are flabby. In reality, we all know very young persons who are sedentary and have high body fat and older persons who exercise reasonably and have great muscle conditioning. It's why the table-driven caliper measurements for body fat are worthless: they assume you have the same level of conditioning as other people your age. We'll talk about this more at the end of this chapter, but in the meantime, take your last look at Table 6 and then throw it away. You should target your ideal body fat, and not decide to be as fat and flabby as others your age.

	AGE			
	20-30	**30-40**	**40-50**	**50-60+**
		<or>		
	ACTIVITY LEVEL			
	v High	**---------->**		**Low**
Men	15-20%	18-23%	20-24%	23-27%
Women	19-25%	20-28%	23-31%	27-34%

Table 6 – Typical ranges for male and female body fat as a function of age or activity.

Table 7 proposes for you a target range for body fat based on your gender. The ranges shown are based on guidelines developed by the *American Council on Exercise*, and should give you insight on the level of body fat **you** should target in determining your ideal weight by the body fat measurement.

To be at a healthy level of fat and weight, you should determine a suitable body fat percentage inside the target range of **Table 7**. Like the evaluation of muscularity in the modified-BMI method, identifying a target inside the range requires a little bit of self-evaluation.

As I mentioned, many references cite the fact that older persons of the same weight carry a higher percentage of body fat than younger persons. While this may be true, it is more an observation of population data than a statement of an objective. Older persons lose muscle mass and gain body fat because they become less active. For men in particular, lower activity and higher body fat leads to lower testosterone level, which further abets the accumulation of corporal fat and deterioration of muscle. If you decide to be active and aggressive with your activities, you can be healthy at the lower end of the target range even as your age advances. This is why Table 7 does not include an age evolution. That would just "enable" you to set low standards and settle for getting fat as you age. That is what you are trying to avoid!

Table 7 suggests a target body fat percentage for men and ("Target Range"). If you decide to be active and like exercise, you can easily elect the lower half of the range even as you age. In the absence of any better judgment, I would suggest you target the midpoint of the range. If you are older than 50, you might target a point or two higher. For a man at 160, the difference between 17% and 14% is about 5 pounds. For a woman at 130, the difference between 23% and 19% is about 6 pounds.

	Essential	Elite Athlete	Target Range	Excess	Very Excessive
Men	4%	6-10%	10-17%	18-27%	27% +
Women	12%	12-15%	15-25%	26-35%	35% +

Table 7 – Body fat objectives: target a level inside the "Target Range".

Calculating your target weight with a target body fat.

Once you have a target body fat percentage, it's time to calculate your ideal weight as follows:

1. Measure your current body fat (*Current BF%* --- instructions on how to get it measured will follow)
2. Use **Table 7** to determine the ideal body fat for your gender, you can pick the midpoint of the target range to establish an initial goal (*Target BF%*)
3. Calculate the your ideal weight using this formula:

$$Ideal\ Weight = (Current\ Weight) \cdot \frac{(1 - Current\ BF\%)}{(1 - Target\ BF\%)} \qquad (Eqn.\ 3)$$

In this equation, "*Current BF%*" is your current body fat (from a measurement) and "*Target BF%*" if your target body fat (from **Table 7**). This formula may look a little more complicated than you expected. You **cannot** simply subtract current and target body fat percentages to get the correct result, because as you lose weight, the same amount of fat represents a higher and higher percentage of your weight (sucks, doesn't it).

Example 1 – A 35 year-old woman who is 5'7" has added 16 pounds over the previous ten years and now weighs 138 pounds. She realizes she is overweight. Even though she exercises regularly, she has developed excess fat on her belly and arms. A precise measurement of her body fat yields a measure of 28%. Since she currently exercises, and plans to increase her level and intensity of exercise to stay in shape, she decides that based on **Table 7** a good target for her is 18% body fat. Using the ideal weight formula, she calculated her final weight at (138 lbs)·(1-.28)/(1-.18) = 121 pounds.

Example 2 – A 42 year-old man has been fat since childhood and has decided he must lose weight for his health. His height is 5'10" and he currently weighs 290 pounds. A precise measurement of his body fat yields a result of 52%. Looking at **Table 7** he decides a good target for him would be 15% body fat. Using the formula for ideal weight based on body fat, he calculates his ideal weight at (290 lbs)·(1-.52)/(1-.15) = 164 pounds.

Example 3 – A 39 year-old 20 has a 42% body fat and weighs 190 pounds. She decides for her health, she needs to get her body fat to the mid-point of the acceptable range – i.e. 20%. Using **(Eqn. 3)** she calculates her target weight: (190 lbs)·(1-.42)/(1-.20) = 138 pounds.

After you calculate your resulting body weight at you target body fat level, you may and say "Shoot, I haven't weighed that much since I was in college." That's exactly what we are going for here.

If you intend to improve your muscle tone and mass as you lose weight, you can eventually add back 5 to 10 pounds generally for men, or 3 to 8 pounds for women. It's very important to have your body fat measured if you are adding muscle, so that there is an honest assessment of lean mass as you near your ideal weight. You wouldn't want muscle mass gains to mask loss of fat. Methods for having your body fat measured are discussed in the next section.

Measuring Your Current Body Fat

Less reliable methods to measure body fat. The most common way to measure your body fat is a so-called **caliper measurement**. This method is the most common because it is the easiest and cheapest method to take a quick measure of body. All you need is a set of calipers and a reference table, and these can be purchased inexpensively online. Many personal trainers use this method because it is easy and requires little equipment **(Figure 3)**. You can also use this method yourself by purchasing an inexpensive set of calipers and tables online.

Caliper measurements are performed by using the caliper tool to measure a number of skin-folds. The thickness of the folds are added together and then, together with your age, used to look up your body fat in a 2-dimensional table.

The tables are built by measuring the actual body fat of thousands of people using one of the more precise methods discussed later, and then populating a table based on the age and caliper measurements of the people who were actually tested precisely. A typical technique for a woman would measure a skin fold on the back of the arm, the thigh, and the hip, and look up the resulting body fat in 3-measure table for women.

The drawback to this approach is *that if your body fat is not the same as the average of all the people measured who have your same total skin-fold measurements and age,* the table will be inaccurate. In fact, the tables show a higher body fat results for the same skin-fold measures as you age. This is because most people, as they age become more sedentary and actually do carry more fat. If you continue to be active and exercise as you age, the tables will be widely inaccurate. A man who is 47 would have a body fat estimate 5 points higher than a man who is 25 for the same skin fold measurements in a typical table. Likewise, if you tend to carry your body fat in areas not tested by the method (for example in the butt for women tested on the thigh and hips) the results will also be widely inaccurate.

Caliper measurements are worthwhile in detecting changes in your body fat. For that reason, if you are a person who is losing your last thirty pounds to reach an ideal weight, but possibly also doing some training to improve muscle, a caliper test performed every week or two can be worthwhile to monitor that you are consistently losing fat. On the other hand, if the caliper measure is the only body fat measurement technique you have access to, I would not use this metric to calculate your ideal body weight as set forth in the previous section, because the absolute number could easily be off by 4 to 5 points, which is an ocean.

For example, suppose you are a woman whose weight is 145 pounds, and your caliper measured body fat is 30%, but your actual body fat is only 25%. You want to move to 20% body fat. The caliper measurement would result in an ideal weight target of 126 pounds when the correct target is 136 pounds.

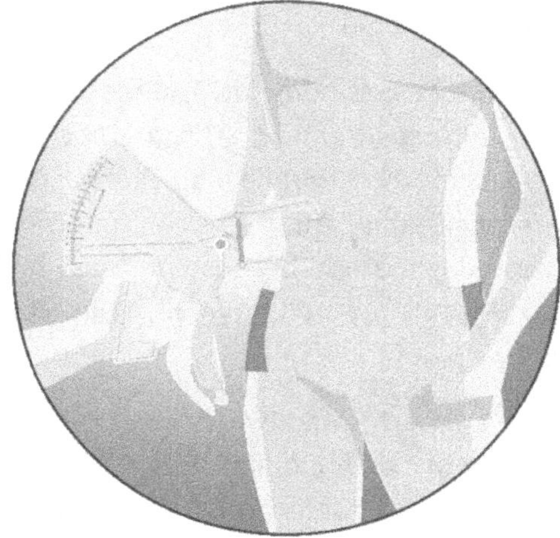

Figure 3 – A caliper used to estimate body fat.

You may have seen scales in pharmacies or retail stores that have electrodes which measure your body fat. This method is called "bioelectrical impedance". Your resistance to the flow of electricity through your body is related to how much fat you carry, and in this method, your impedance is compared to those of the same age, weight, and gender on a statistical basis. This method has the same drawbacks as a caliper approach, and should only be used to monitor changes in body fat. It is not as an absolute indicator or a metric that should be used to calculate ideal weight using (Eqn. 3).

Accurate measures of body fat. There are two ways to accurately measure your body fat. One method is called **hydrostatic testing**. The other is called **Air Displacement Plethysmography**. In both hydrostatic testing and air displacement plethysmography the objective is to calculate the overall density of your body and then to use that to calculate your body fat.

In **hydrostatic testing**, your body fat is calculated via immersion: you are weighed in water and on dry land. Since the density of water is known, how much you weigh in water compared to how much you weigh on dry land can easily be used to calculate your density relative to the density of water. Density is usually expressed in grams per cubic centimeter (g/cm^3). The density of fat tissue is also well known, as is the density of the non-fat part of your body (bone, blood, organs, fluids). Once your overall density is calculated by the water weigh-in, the percentage of fat is calculated by identifying the combination of fat at its low density, and everything else at its higher density that results in your observed density.

Hydrostatic testing is not perfect. First, the density of "everything else" that is not fat in the body can vary slightly from person to person, although it have been verified in a narrow range by thousands of observations. The riskier part of the calculation is a correction that needs to be made for the volume of air that might remain in your lungs while you are being weighed underwater. All that said, research has suggested that hydrostatic testing is generally accurate to within about 0.5 percentage points in body fat measurement. Caliper measures can see errors of 5 points or more in certain cases.

Air Displacement Plethysmography uses a different method to measure your overall density. You are placed in a "pod" of known volume. The volume of the pod is reduced slightly and the change in air pressure inside the pod is measured. How sharply pressure increases tells the operator the remaining volume of air in the bod after you got in. With your volume calculated this way, plus your weight on dry land, it easy to calculate your density. With your density, the calculation or your body fat proceeds just as in the calculation for hydrostatic weighing. Possibilities for inaccuracy are similar except the plethysmography method seems to naturally handle the issue of the air in your lungs, so it has the potential to work better than hydrostatic weighing. Again research suggests this method can be accurate to within 0.5 points.

If you have the opportunity, I recommend you get a body fat measurement at the outset of your decision to reach your ideal weight using either hydrostatic testing or air displacement. These two methods are accurate, and give you a set goal for ideal weight at the beginning of your effort. You can calculate your ideal weight with a body fat target and compare it to the approach using BMI, or average the two objectives. As you near your ideal weight, you can be re-tested and you'll be able to adjust your final weight if you are adding muscle while reaching a body fat objective.

You should be able to find a center for a hydrostatic body fat measurement or an air displacement measurement online or by calling a local health club. The commercial name for air displacement testing is "Body Pod", and these tests can be taken for $50 or less.

Glycogen Water

Earlier in this chapter I said that for purposes of losing weight, your body is "fat" and "everything else", and you only lose weight by losing fat. I also said there was a "big footnote" to this simplification. That footnote is on the topic of water weight, or *glycogen water*.

Our body packs energy stores that it wants to have available for immediate use in the form of a "glycogen". Glycogen is stored in the liver and in the muscles. Each gram of glycogen requires an additional 2.7 grams of water to facilitate that storage. That can lead to pretty hefty glycogen weight. As a result, if you are eating more calories than you need, especially if you eat a lot of carbs, which are readily available sources of glycogen for the body, you may have 5 to 7 pounds or more (in some persons 15 to 20 pounds!) of this so-called "glycogen water" stored in your liver and other tissues. This is the weight that has for years been called "water weight". The nature of it has been much better understood as the result of recent research.

Persons who go on a low carbohydrate diet will lose this glycogen weight fairly quickly. That's why you often hear persons getting on low carb diets say they "lost a lot of weight right away". This is not fat loss. When you are at your ideal weight, if you choose to eat a low-carb or paleo diet, you will not carry a lot of glycogen or water weight, and in that case your final ideal weight may be lower than indicated by body fat objectives.

Glycogen weight leaves quickly on a change of diet, especially a low-carb diet, but it can also come back quickly after a great big meal or binge-ful holiday weekend. All you have to do is gorge yourself with a lot of carbs and it can all come back in a couple of days. Stepping on the scale frequently, you'll get a better handle on this effect. I urge you not to get too distracted by it either. Your goal is to lose fat. I'm not going to tell you to go on a permanent no-carbs diet. Even Dr. Atkins didn't do that. As a result, water weight will come and go. Based on your dietary cycle. If you do decide to discipline yourself with a permanent low-carbohydrate diets, it's an additional opportunity to permanently reduce your weight.

SOME NOTES FOR THE REALLY FAT

A lot of discussion in this chapter has centered on getting a very narrow fix on your ideal weight to the last pound. If you are fat or obese, and have a 100 pounds to lose, you may be wondering why you are reading this book. "Why am I worrying about whether a BMI measures tells me I should be 170 and a body-fat measure says I should weigh 175? I'm 300 pounds for God's sake."

To keep you motivated as we move into Chapters Chapter 4 to Chapter 8 on **how** to reach your ideal weight I want to make a couple of contextual comments. First, as we discussed earlier in this chapter, you can't succeed at anything if you don't set the right goal. For weight loss, the goal at the outset should be the correct finish line. If you are 300 pounds, and say, "My goal is to see if I can lose 15 pounds," you might lose 15 pounds, but then, you'll find an excuse to rest, compromise, or wait for a reason to lose the next 15 – shit you've proven now you can lose 15 – meanwhile often adding back 10 or 20 pounds. I need to put you on a steady, relentless walk to your ideal weight. Once you understand the dynamics, you'll enjoy the journey and even more so the final destination.

Next, the reason it is important to identify your ideal weight at the outset is that you might think of weight loss as two phases. The process of losing the weight does not change between the phases, but the impact does. If you weigh 300 pounds, you might say "I'd be thrilled to get to 190 pounds and hold that weight", but if your ideal weight is 160 pounds, there are a couple of problems with this view:

- you are still overweight if you are 30 pounds overweight;
- many health and social dividends come in the last 30 pounds of weight loss.

With respect to the second bullet, if you really weigh 300 pounds, there are tremendous health dividends to losing that first 110 pounds; however there are still many health risks – diabetes, cancer, high blood pressure that persist when are 30 pounds overweight. Finally, a great deal of the sense of energy, optimism, and well-being comes with the last 30 pounds.

Now let's suppose you've been at 190 pounds for a long time, and your ideal weight is 160 pounds (without adding back muscle which you might decide to do). For persons in this group, I've found that if you ask them if they need to lose weight, they will often agree that they could lose 10 or 15 pounds. The under-appreciation of the correct weight is extremely common for persons who are 15% overweight. Even persons who focus on BMI are often misled. The CDC standard for healthy BMI used to be 27, now its 25, and many people are overweight at 25. So if you are in this group, you may have picked up this book because you want to lose 15 pounds. I'm selling you on the reality that it is super important for you to take an open-eyed calculation of how much you really should weigh and set the right goal at the outset. Again, a lot of the dividends for you will come in the last 20 pounds you lose, not the first 10.

Exercises – Chapter 2 How to Calculate Your Ideal Weight

You may want a calculator. Completing these exercises will help you plan for reaching your ideal weight.

1. Calculate your BMI ...

My weight in pounds =	
My height in inches =	
My BMI = weight / (height x height) x 703	
My BMI = [_______ / (_______ x_______)] x 703 =	

2. Evaluate Yourself – What is your ideal weight?

A. Use **Table 3** to evaluate your **muscularity**. How do you rate yourself 1 to 6? _______

B. Use **Table 5** to determine your ideal weight. In the box for your gender, pick the column for your self-evaluated muscularity. Run your finger down the page to the row with your height. The value in that row and that column is your ideal weight. Write it in the box.

Ideal ☐ Weight

3. Use the body-fat method to check your work (Only if you can get access to an accurate body fat measurement location!).

A. Look at **Table 7**. How aggressive do you want to be? Pick a body-fat percentage in the target range for your gender. Write it down!

————

B. If you choose, locate a "body pod" center near you. Have your body fat accurately measured. What is your body fat today? **(DO NOT USE A CALIPER METHOD!)**

————

C. Calculate your ideal weight based on target body fat. In the formula, write your body fat as a decimal, not a percentage.

My weight (pounds) =	
My target body fat (%) =	
My current body fat (%) =	
Ideal weight = **My weight X** **(1-current body fat) / (1 – target body fat)**	
Ideal weight = ______ X (1 - ___) /(1 - ___) =	

Chapter 3 – How to Determine Your Ideal Calories

In this Chapter I start to provide the knowledge you need to reach your ideal weight: a sense of how much you can eat. In determining how much you can eat, counting both the calories coming in (what you ate), and the calories going out (the energy you used) are important to understand if you've created the energy deficit needed to lose weight. In actual practice, these numbers are hard to measure very precisely every single day; however, it's important for you to have reasonable sense of their magnitude so that you can calibrate your eating habits to a practical everyday reality.

The Axiom of Energy Balance

I want to talk about the inescapable axiom of energy balance and weight, because this knowledge will help you to reduce all the dietary information and advice you find in the world to basic elements of eating calories and using calories. The objective is to help you understand that diet systems and methods which are honest drive you to one goal: reducing one and increasing the other.

Those sadistic enough to have studied engineering realize you deal with a lot of flowing systems that include moving liquid, gases, and heat. They always teach you do draw a dotted line around your system, and then count everything that comes in or out, and that will give you the future state of your system. For example, if **Figure 4** is a system of flowing water, and the dotted circle is my "system boundary", I may want to know at some point in the future how much water will be in that tank. If I know how much water is in the tank now, and I know the rate it is flowing in via Pipe A, and the rate it is flowing out via Pipe B, I can calculate the amount of water that will be in the tank at some future point in time.

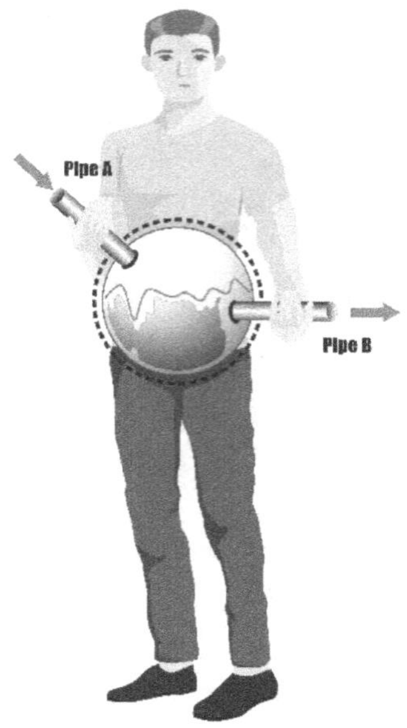

Figure 4 – A basic engineering mass balance.

Your body has a similar basic "calorie" balance. If you know your initial weight, you know how many calories you take in, and you know how many calories you expend, you can calculate your future weight (**Figure 5**).

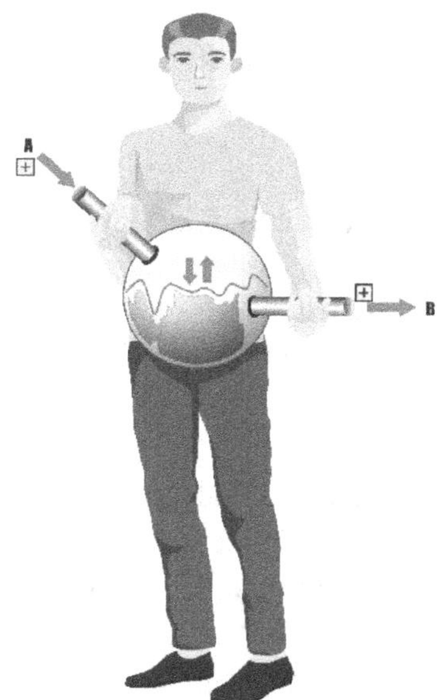

Figure 5 – Your body weight as an engineering balance.

Given that most engineering systems aren't as simple as Figure 4 – many have both liquids and gases that can be compressed, heat sources, and chemical reactions that can affect the future state of the system.   All that stuff has to be calculated, tracked separately and transfers between states and phases have to be calculated and tracked.

In the same vein, your body isn't actually as simple as Figure 5. Food turns into certain sugars or proteins, then into immediate energy or maybe fat, and back to energy via a variety of paths. (Kevin D Hall, 2011), "Quantification of the effect of energy imbalance on body weight" is a fantastic reference if you are interested in the interplay between fat tissue, lean tissue, glycogen water, cellular water, and energy balance".)

Despite the underlying complexity, the simplified representation of Figure 5 is complete and comprehensive in terms of outcomes when you translate both food, body fat, and activity to the common units of energy (the calorie is a unit of energy). You have an initial weight today ("my weight today"). You have a daily caloric intake. And you have a daily energy expenditure. A pound of fat is manufactured by your body from 3,500 excess calories. The difference between your energy consumption and energy expenditure is your weight gain (or lose) over any period of time. In fact, for every roughly 3,500 calories you consume in excess of what you expend, you'll gain about one pound of fat. Conversely for losing pounds.

To calculate how many calories you can eat, you need to know how many you expend. Your daily energy expenditure has two parts your "resting metabolic rate" ("RMR") which is about 1,200 to 1,800 calories per day depending on size and gender, plus extra calories that you expend doing your daily activities ("ACTIVITY").   RMR describes the calories you use for a beating heart, breathing, organ function, and metabolism. In other words, it's the calories you would burn if you sat around and did absolutely nothing but breathe.

As I said, for every 3,500 calories you take in ("my Calories Consumed") in excess of what you expend ("my RMR plus ACTIVITY") you will gain one pound of fat. That's right: a pound of fat stores 3,500 calories of energy for your later use.

Figure 5 is subtly more complex than Figure 4. Figure 4 is about water mass or weight. Figure 5 is framed in terms of the fat-mass of an energy equivalent. That's irrelevant. The simplification is accurate and complete. It does not matter how much the food you eat weighs. If it contains 3,500 unexpended calories it will be converted by your body to a pound of fat, and you will poop out the rest.

This is a key point when you think about diet tools and aids: *for every 3,500 calories you consume in excess of what you expend, you'll gain a pound of fat. For every 3,500 calories of energy you expend in excess of what you eat, you'll lose a pound of fat.* Diet plans that tell you that you can eat more and lose weight are generally lying, unless they have some definition of food quantity not anchored in calories (size of the food?), or unless they are going to advise you run for an hour for each candy bar you consume.

How Much Can I Eat? – A Discrete Formula

So how much can I eat in order to reach my ideal weight? There are really two answers – how much to eat while you are losing weight, and how much to eat after you've reached your ideal weight.

While you are losing weight, you need to create a calorie / energy deficit. The most practical approach to losing weight is targeting to lose one pound per week. A pound of fat, after it is metabolized (consumed by the body for energy) releases 3,500 calories of energy. In order to lose a pound of fat in a week, you need to expend 3,500 more calories in energy than you eat.

If you count calories, this means on average, you need to burn 500 calories more per day than you eat (500 calories / day * 7 days / week = 3,500 calories per week). Well shit, then the next question is, "How many calories per day do I burn?"

As we discussed, your daily caloric expenditure is composed of two elements: Your RMR and your ACTIVITY (walking, running, moving, biking, etc.).

If we really wanted to use a precise method to measure your RMR, we would have to place you in a giant calorimeter (a very precise instrument for measuring heat) for a day while you rest comfortably. To know your ACTIVITY, we'd have to precisely analyze your activities, or follow you with that calorimeter, knowing all the while that the quantity and intensity of those activities could vary widely between the day we checked and other days. So bottom line what I'm saying is that there is no analog to hydrostatic testing for fat measurement that is an easy, reliable, and affordable proxy in accurately measuring your daily caloric consumption.

Fortunately, while this daily caloric usage is hard to measure precisely, it's easy to estimate accurately, due to decades of research and measurement on test subjects.

The following formula governs your daily energy balance:

$$Balance = Calories\ (Consumed) - RMR - ACTVITY \qquad (Eqn.\ 4)$$

Balance can be positive or negative. If your calorie expenditures (RMR and ACTIVITY) are more than what you eat, your balance is negative, and you are losing weight. If your calories consumed on the other hand exceeds what you expend, your balance is positive, and you are gaining weight. If you aim to lose one pound a week, you need a balance of -500 calories per day. On this basis, you can calculate your allowable daily calories by this formula, where I am using -500 for *"Balance"* and replacing the term *"Calories (Consumed)"* with *"Calories (Allowed)"*.

$$Calories\ (Allowed) = RMR + ACTIVITY - 500 \qquad \text{(Eqn. 5)}$$

Easy!

But we need an estimate for your RMR and activity to get an answer. How do you estimate your RMR? RMR is related to your size and your gender. It's related to your size because workload on your heart and workload of organ function is related to your size. Men burn more in RMR than women, because they carry more muscle, and muscle uses energy while resting. These gender-based formulas should estimate your RMR:

$$RMR_{male} = \frac{Current\ Weight\ [lbs] \cdot 24}{2.2} \qquad \text{(Eqn. 6)}$$

$$RMR_{female} = \frac{Current\ Weight\ [lbs] \cdot 0.9 \cdot 24}{2.2} \qquad \text{(Eqn. 7)}$$

These correlations are pretty good for most people. They are based on collecting data from large numbers of people (Marie Dunford, 2015). If you are very heavy – 50 pounds or more overweight – these formulas may overstate your RMR somewhat.

If you are in this category, you have two options which will yield similar results: (1) calculate your RMR at your current weight and calculate it at your ideal weight and average the two measurements; (2) calculate your RMR using this gender neutral correlation for fat people:

$$RMR_{m\ or\ f} = \frac{1.3 \cdot (1 - Current\ BF\%) \cdot Current\ Weight\ [lbs] \cdot 24}{2.2} \qquad \text{(Eqn. 8)}$$

This estimation above requires you to have a good estimate of your body fat percentage. Hopefully you got it checked after you read Chapter 2. If you are using the BMI table to calculate your ideal weight and haven't had the chance to have your body fat measured, just use the first method above: but calculate your RMR at both your (1) current weight and (2) ideal weight and average the two measures.

Just as I mentioned there are precise ways to measure body fat (immersion and Air Displacement Plethysmography), there are more precise methods to measure your resting metabolic rate. Typically this involves wearing a mask and measuring your usage of oxygen over a 10 or 15 minute sample period. Such tests can be found at reasonable cost, but are not widely available, and the issue is that your "sample period" might not be representative of your average resting metabolism over the course of the day while reading, working at your desk, sleeping, watching TV, etc. Shoot, you could be nervous when you take the test and impact the results.

As I suggested with the alternate formula for heavy people, your RMR does change as you lose weight. Your fat doesn't use a lot of energy when you are resting – not as much as lean tissue – but it uses some. Also if you are heavy, your heart and organs work harder. If you are interested in understanding this science better, the scholarly paper "Quantification of the effect of energy imbalance on bodyweight" (Hall, et al, *Lancet,* 2011) has an excellent discussion of how your RMR may vary as you lose weight, and also in an appendix provides a mathematical model of human metabolism that approximates the effect. A great resource if you are a geeky-science type. Otherwise the approximations of either **(Eqn.** 6) or **(Eqn.** 7) will suit your purpose just fine.

While I stressed the value of accurate body fat measurements in Chapter 2, the correlations based on your weight are probably sufficient for estimating your daily calories. Just remember, if you are very fat, use the correlation based on body fat percentage ((Eqn. 8)), or the average of your RMR at your current fatty weight (using (Eqn. 8)) and your ideal weight (using either (Eqn. 6) or (Eqn. 7) depending on gender).

OK, so how do you estimate your ACTIVITY? Your calories burned by your daily exercise and activities are usually actually less than your RMR. Unless you are extremely active, beating your heart and running your organs is the most active thing you do. You can estimate your ACTIVITY expenditure based on your RMR if you can make an honest self-assessment of how active you are.

Table 8 shows you how to calculate your ACTIVITY based on your RMR which you just calculated. To use the figure, first read the descriptions of the activity levels and decide where you fit. Multiply the number in the table by your calculated RMR and you'll have an estimate of the calories you use every day in your activities. If you think you don't quite fit in a table row – suppose you are more than "sedentary" but less than "low active", you can interpolate halfway between the number in each of those two rows.

Activity Level	ACTIVITY Male	ACTIVITY Female	Comments
Sedentary	0.28 · RMR	0.24 · RMR	Mostly seated or standing daily living activities; no exercise or other active leisure activities.
Low Active	0.51 · RMR	0.52 · RMR	Light exercise and leisure activites (i.e. walking 50 minutes per day or golfing 40 minutes per day).
Active	0.74 · RMR	0.74 · RMR	Moderate exercise and leisure activities (i.e. cycling moderately 75 minutes per day or playing tennis 90 minutes per day).
Very Active	1.08 · RMR	1.07 · RMR	Heavy manual labor job or heavy exercise and leisure activities (i.e. jogging 75 minutes per day or playing basketball 60 minutes per day).

Table 8 – Tool to estimate your daily ACTIVITY calories based on RMR.

Once you've decided where you best fit in **Table 8** its time to calculate your daily allowed calories for losing one pound per week using **(Eqn.** 5).

Example – A woman who weighs 165 pounds is 35 pounds overweight based on her ideal weight. She wants to calculate her allowable daily calories so that she can reach her ideal weight in about 35 weeks. Since she is not ridiculously fat (not more than 50 pounds above ideal weight) she uses the correlation for female RMR to estimate her resting metabolic rate at (165*0.9*24/2.2) = 1,620 calories. The woman has a desk job that is basically sedentary. She does play indoor soccer three times a week, but she is only out on the field about 20 minutes in a typical game. She figures that she is somewhere between "Sedentary" and "Low Active" on the table in **Table 8**. As a result she uses "0.38" as her multiplier of RMR to calculate her ACTIVITY (half way between 0.24 and 0.52). Since her RMR is 1,620, her ACTIVITY is approximately 0.38 * 1,620 = 615 calories. Her average daily energy expenditures is 2,235 calories. Since she wants to lose a pound per week, she uses the *Calories (Allowed)* formula to calculate her daily allowable consumption = 1,620 + 615 – 500 = 1,736 calories.

Ironically, calculating how many calories you eat is fairly easy if you are conscientious. Online apps such as *"MyFitnessPal"* are extremely exhaustive in foods they cover and very easy to use. Knowing your RMR and activity expenditure is the harder part. Knowing how much you eat doesn't do you much good if you don't know how much you burn. We don't know your precise RMR and we could be off by a 100 to 200 calories. That is a lot when you need to ensure a deficit of 500 calories per day. .

That being said, the *Calories (Allowed)* formula is a great estimate of your average daily allowed calories over the term of weeks and months, even if it is flawed on a particular day. It's a number you need to know and be aware of. It puts the decisions you make around consumption into a context you can start to feel comfortable with

("Should I eat 1,000 calories at Chipotle this meal?"). If you are concerned about overestimating what you are allowed to eat, move yourself up one row in the ACTIVITY calculation and calculate your allowable calories again. That will provide you a reliable target range.

Typing everything you eat into a calorie database on the web and recording it is not practical for most people. Our objective here is to get you close to the right numbers so you can develop good instincts. The impact of your overall level of eating on weight will reveal itself in your experience. A 1,300 calorie quick serve restaurant meal should give you pause when you are targeting 1,750 calories per day. You can't do that every day at work. You can do it occasionally. Later, I'll also discuss the importance of frequent weighing to monitor and develop your instincts around progress. Very few people have the time and compulsiveness to assiduously count calories indefinitely. Even if you have that determination, your conclusions are susceptible to the least accurate part of the *Calories (Allowed)* formula, which is your RMR and ACTIVITY.

Fitness bracelets, such as Jawbone and Fitbit have become very popular for estimating your calories burned. Unfortunately they aren't more accurate than the methods in this chapter. A *Wall Street Journal* articles cited several studies suggesting that these devices are usually off by 15- to 20% (McGinty, 2015). A device that overestimates your calories burned by 10% would cause you to gain about 2 pounds per month, while giving you the false assurance that you should be maintaining weight at a fixed level.

By weighing yourself frequently, and understanding those daily and weekly measurements in the context of your eating and activity, you start to create a feedback loop that will deliver an intuitive sense of cause and effect. You'll learn to adjust your behavior accordingly. I'll talk more about the importance of frequent weighing in Chapter 8.

Exercises – Chapter 3 *How to Determine Your Calories*

1. Let's estimate how many calories you can eat every day. First we'll calculate how many calories you burn just sitting doing nothing (your "resting metabolic rate" or RMR)

MEN:	[WEIGHT] x 24 ÷ 2.2	
My RMR= [ ] x 24 ÷ 2.2		=
WOMEN:	[WEIGHT] x 24 x 0.9 ÷ 2.2	
My RMR= [ ] x 24 x 0.9 ÷ 2.2	=	

Resting Metabolic Rate (Daily Calories Burned Sitting Still)

2. Next, we'll add the approximate calories you burn with your activities.

A. Use **Table 8** from this chapter to honestly evaluate your ACTIVITY for your gender. (Most of us are not better than "sedentary". If you exercise daily for less than an hour, you are low sedentary.) Your factor is the number in the table for your gender (ranging from 0.24 to 1.08).

B. Calculate your **ACTIVITY** calories by multiplying the factor from **Table 8** by your resting metabolic rate from Step 1 above:

My ACTIVITY = My RMR x (Table 8 Factor)

My ACTIVITY = [   ] x [   ] =

Daily Calories Burned by Your Activity (Daily Calories)

3. Next we'll calculate your total allowed calories to maintain your current weight:

ALLOWED = My RMR + My ACTIVITY

ALLOWED = [   ] + [   ] =

Total Calories Burned by You Each Day

4. If you want to lose a pound a week, you need to reduce those calories by around 500 per day:

ALLOWED (1lb) = My RMR + My ACTIVITY − 500

ALLOWED (1Lb) = [   ] + [   ] − 500 =

Daily Calories Allowed to Lose 1 Pound per Week

Chapter 4 – Hunger

In this chapter, I am going to start to give a basic tools to reach your ideal weight.

The greatest economist ever to toil in the "dismal science", a man named Milton Friedman, said "Inflation is always and everywhere a monetary phenomenon…" In that spirit there is a similar truism related to waistline inflation: "Obesity is everywhere and always a hunger phenomenon". Ultimately reaching your ideal weight is about knowing how to conquer hunger. A $70 B industry for supplements and diet aids in the United States can be reduced substantially to a war on hunger. But what if we are fighting the war the wrong way, or what if we are fighting the wrong war?

This chapter is organized to give you first a background on "obesity as a hunger phenomenon". I'll provide a brief discussion on how systems, diets, products, pharmaceuticals, and interventions seek to address hunger, so that you can put these in context. Next I'll talk about how hunger and food addiction have evolved in first-world societies, helping you to understand the context that causes you to succumb to a food addiction. Finally, I'll give you the tools and information you need to beat hunger and eat the correct amount of food. This is a battle that's winnable. You have to decide to win and then you have to win with my help.

Hunger is the only enemy of your reaching your ideal weight. It's the only impulse that cues you to eat – and to eat too much. Nearly all diet programs and aids boil down to helping (or claiming to help) you deal with the hunger that comes naturally from eating the correct amount of food. When you view the problem this way, it can lead you to confront and conquer the problem, without the distraction of programs and processes that promise to get you something for nothing. Your sense of hunger is an urge that lies to you. It will not lead you to eat the correct amount of food. As I wrap up this chapter, we'll discuss the process of your taking direct accountability for what you eat, and I will deliver coping strategies that will be expanded in the following chapter, enabling you to control the demon of hunger.

DIET PLANS, SCHEMES, AIDS, AND SUPPLEMENTS: BOILING IT DOWN TO HUNGER

Since your weight is strictly related to how many calories you consume and how many you burn (*RMR + ACTIVITY*), it should be clear where this takes us in terms of fighting fatness and reaching ideal weight. The mission to conquer your weight is a mission on conquering hunger. I'm going to help you and empower you to do that. For context, I'll spend the next few paragraphs talking about diet plans and aids and putting them in context of how they help you address hunger.

The systems, methods, tools, supplements, diets, and routines are part of a $70 B US annual diet and fitness industry. Reaching your ideal weight is about eating the correct amount of food (calories). Succumbing to hunger prevents you from succeeding. Nearly all programs and methods to help you lose weight boil down to helping you deal with hunger. Those that are legitimate and sincere give you tools and support. Those that are deceptive make unrealistic make untrue promises.

If you have the impression that I am about to advise you not to use any commercial diet products, you are incorrect. Reaching your ideal weight is about eating the correct amount of food. Not everyone will enjoy the exact same sources of inspiration and motivation. My goal is not to sell you an alternative to established products and systems, or tell you not to purchase them. It's to help you put them in context.

My goals so far are the following:

- Teach you how to calculate your ideal weight (done!)
- Teach you the correct amount of food calories to reach your ideal weight (done!)
- Teach you how to deal with hunger to ensure you reach your ideal weight (coming)
- Ensure you reach the best health, optimism, and sense of well-being that you have the potential to achieve (coming)

Those diet aids that are intellectually honest may help you with motivation, with focus on the correct amount of food to eat, and they may just generally help you get through those days when you are eating less. On the other hand, if you place responsibility on these programs for success, and take responsibility out of your own hands, you will fail.

Just like a cup of coffee or your favorite TV show helps you get through your day, diet programs and aids may help you get through your day. ***Absolutely nothing wrong with that***. According to participants in the *National Weight Control Registry*, which we'll discuss more in Chapter 8, about half of us who are successful at losing substantial weight and keeping it off for five years, used some kind of assistive product or program, and half of us do not. The greatest risks to your success occur when you turn responsibility for success over to these methods or programs. "If I just follow this program precisely, it will deliver the result it promises." This is almost never true and it removes your accountability from the equation. It is a cop-out. Only you will make your success and you have to be responsible for it.

If you look objectively at the weight-loss industry (excluding exercise programs and routines), you will conclude that nearly all legitimate plans, schemes, aids, and supplement programs can be reduced to helping you confront hunger. The only possible exception to this formalism is products focused very narrowly on calorie counting. Calorie counting products may help you monitor your daily calories without providing any support, inspiration, methods, or promises about conquering hunger or any suggestions on what you should do when you've reached your food quota and you are still hungry.

Table 9, shows you a broad classification of all the types of weight management tools that are in the industry, and how they aim to help you deal with hunger. Certain brands use more than one approach or method to achieving the same goal (a good example being *Weight Watchers*).

Category	Examples	Target	Comments
Moral Support, Motivation, Encouragement	*Weight Watchers, MediFast, Weight Loss Buddy*	hunger	helps the dieters avoid tempation to eat more than correct quantity of food
Diet Books and Plans - Legitimate	*8-hour Diet, Every other Day Diet, South Beach Diet*	hunger	provide good advice about diet, eating, actionable methods, motivation, support
Diet Books and Plans - Deceptive	*Many*	hunger	deceptive plans often assert you can lose weight by eating certain type of food, or can diet, eating as much as you want, or *without feeling hungry*
Prescription Appetite Supressants	*Belviq, Saxenda*	hunger	no magic bullet yet, several close to market, safety and side effects to consider
Gastric Bypass Surgery	*Many primary care hospitals and programs throughout US*	hunger	not the magic bullet once thought - as patients often defeat surgery years later - patient still must show lifestyle and willpower forever
Diet Supplements	*Many*	hunger	always deceptive or fraudulent or not effective
Calorie Counting Aids	*Deal-a-Meal, MyFitnessPal*	food quantity	only category of diet aid that doesn't necessarily have a claim about hunger management
Retail Diet Food and Subscription Programs	*Weight Watchers, Medifast, freshdiet, BistroMD*	hunger / food quantity	may help you limit your food quantity if you are disciplined, usually have claims on hunger

Table 9 – Nearly all weight loss aids focus on helping you deal with hunger.

My intent in writing this book is to distill for you what it means to lose weight --- completely unanchored from all the methods, systems, and self-help that are designed to help you lose weight. I am going to make the assertion here that there isn't anything wrong with any of these tools, whether you like "Weight Watchers" – which is a system of calorie-aware food and moral support, or "The 8-hour Diet" which tells you when to eat, or "The Mediterranean Diet" – which tells you what to eat.

The exception to this pledge not to "disparage" diet aids and programs of course does not apply to books and supplements that make **false or deceptive promises**, or the medical interventions (**drugs** and **surgery**), which may be worthwhile, but which are important enough to bear further discussion.

On deception and hucksterism. There are some diet approaches and supplements that lie to you or make untrue promises to get your attention and money. Here is a brief sampling of some top-selling diet books from Amazon on a recent day:

- "The Fast Metabolism Diet: Eat More Food and Lose More Weight" – *likely deceptive, depends on the definition of "food". If it's based on calories, you'll get fatter if you eat more food, unless you increase exercise more than you increase food.*
- "The Zero Belly Diet: Lose up to 16 Pounds in 14 days" – *short term weight loss can often be achieved by reducing carbs which reduces water weight. Real loss of fat won't reliably (and shouldn't) occur at the rate of more than about one to two pounds per week.*
- "Smoothies for Weight Loss: Delicious Smoothies that Crush Cravings, Fight Fat, and Keep You Thin" – *net metabolism of fat is not caused by any particular food. It's only caused by a negative energy balance: expending more calories than you consume ((Eqn. 5)). While some foods may crush cravings as you eat them, you will always need tools to deal with hunger if you are planning to eat fewer calories than you burn.*
- "How to Lose Belly Fat Fast for Men and Women" – *your body will decide what fat it harvests when you create an energy deficit. Most observations support the idea that the last fat added is usually the first fat burned. There is no credible means to target a particular region of your body for fat metabolism. This is why reaching an ideal weight is important – it ensures your level of fat everywhere will be suitable and attractive.*

I have not read these books, so my comments are only on the titles of the books, and intended only to give you a sense of danger around false promises which are very common in the weight loss industry. The titles above were five of the first seven titles that appeared when I made an Amazon search. My point is that you don't have to look very far to find diet help that is fanciful, false, or misleading. No wonder so many try so hard to so little effect. As a disclaimer, these titles may be intended to get you to purchase a book, and it is possible that these books are better than their titles.

On supplements and pills that claim to cause you to lose weight, I won't wade into providing you any examples. Unfortunately no supplement that makes claims about causing weight loss works, despite the claims of clinical trials that are on all of those bottles. Many contain patently fraudulent claims. These claims are easy to make because the assertions made for over-the-counter supplements are not regulated. There is no persuasive evidence that any over-the-counter supplement except caffeine has any potential to impact weight.

Caffeine is the only possible exception. Taking caffeine won't necessarily cause you to lose weight, but as an exception, it may help you reduce hunger. (Nicotine and other stimulants can have the same impact as caffeine, but due to the much more devastating potential health impacts of using them, only caffeine is addressed further here.)

Of course FDA-approved pharmaceuticals are also another matter, and we'll talk about these shortly.

All non-medical diet programs and aids that are legitimate ultimately are there to provide you with motivation and support to deal with the villain of hunger which is *of necessity* if you are losing or maintaining weight. Those that are honest will tell you they will help you deal with diet and hunger. Those that are dishonest will tell you they can help you lose weight **without hunger**, or with limited sacrifice.

Pharmaceutical solutions. Pharmaceutical interventions are one of two topics, along with gastric surgery, that deserve more discussion. For years there have been rumors and hopes of a legitimate pharmaceutical diet pill, prescribed by a doctor, that will help you lose weight, and for years, that promise has been just over the horizon. If you are one of those people that have always wished you could just "take a pill" to stop your hunger, you may finally be in luck. Several new pharmaceuticals are being approved by the US FDA around 2015 and are hitting the market in the near term.

The first notable FDA-approved pharmaceutical to treat obesity was the "fen-phen" drug combination sold by Wyeth Pharmaceuticals. The drug combo was first marketed widely in 1996. It caused mitral valve (heart) damage so quickly and persuasively, especially in women, that several persons died within months. The drug was taken off the market before the end of 1997, but not before creating $13 B in legal liability for Wyeth. Another drug, Merida, was pulled by Abbott in 2010 because it increased risk of heart attack and stroke in patients.

These tragedies created a more cautious environment for considering safety and efficacy for weight-loss pharmaceuticals, and they created enhanced scrutiny at the FDA. Nevertheless, four drugs have been approved or neared approval recently – Qsymia, Belviq, Contrave, and Saxenda.. These drugs work by a variety of different mechanisms to help you feel less hungry.

These drugs are almost certainly safer than predecessors. That being said, in considering taking a pill to help you with your weight, there are a number of things you should consider. The FDA, while having approved these pills, is requiring continuing long-term safety studies. All of the drugs have been associated with at least one possible "scary" side effect. One of them is connected to a suspicion of thyroid tumors. One is connected to birth-defects. One is under continuing monitoring for increased risk of breast cancer, and several are being monitored for effects on cardiovascular health. For these reasons, doctors are cautious about prescribing them for mild cases of overweight, or for cases that don't include an imminent obesity-caused disease (diabetes, cardiovascular disease, etc.). Insurance may not pay for them if your BMI is not over 30 (that's over 200 pounds if you are 5'9"), or it may not pay form them at all, putting you on the hook for $200 or $300 per month out of pocket.

For your purposes, you should consider the drugs as an aid to possibly help you deal with the demon of hunger as you lose weight. They may help, but you have to decide whether you need that help or whether you'd rather learn to confront hunger on your own ... considering both the cost of the medicine and the risk of taking a pill for the rest of your life that may have long-term health impact. Many people think, "I'll just take the drug til I reach the correct wait and then stop". That never works. Once you stop taking the medicine, if you haven't learned how to deal with hunger, you'll immediately start gaining back the weight you lost. If you don't plan to take the pill forever you are only deferring your inevitable confrontation with hunger. Beating hunger on your own is more rewarding and more permanent than doing it with drugs. Dr. Ronald Sha, director at Duke University's Diet and Fitness Center said "[the drugs] are effective only with lifestyle changes." (Loftus, 2015). If you make the reasonable lifestyle changes we discuss in this book (eating the correct amount of food, tolerating hunger, fasting, moderate exercise), you'll quickly figure out that those pharmaceuticals are extraneous.

If you do decide to use drugs, and then phase them out after meeting a goal, those necessary lifestyle changes will remain your responsibility, and you will find yourself less equipped to deal with them without a pharmaceutical crutch. I am going to talk more about this topic in Chapter 8– Putting it All Together. But what it is important to say now is that the required lifestyle changes, after you have adjusted to them, actually make food more rewarding, and improve your sense of well-being, optimism, and quality of life. ***Nothing wrong with that.*** It's something you should want to do anyway. So you should not see these changes as "scary challenges that you need drugs to confront", but a paradigm shift that will move you to a better life.

If after finishing reading "On Fridays We Fast", you think these pharmaceuticals will give you a needed motivation and boost, then try them under medical supervision. The most important thing is that you not view them as a magic bullet. That perspective will doom you to failure. By the time you're finished here, you'll understand that the change required (and also desired) is ultimately the same for those who may take these drugs and those who don't.

Gastric surgery:

Gastric surgery has become considerably more tolerable and tremendously more prevalent in the United States over the past two decades than it had been before the early 1990's. This is driven not only by the "obesity epidemic" but also by increased experience and ease with the underlying surgery, and marketing by hospitals and health systems to increase volumes of these procedures. Surgery has become more tolerable because even complex bypass surgeries that involve removing large portions of the stomach and intestines can be done laparoscopically, and the laparoscopic band surgery ("lap band"), which does not involve removal of any portion of the stomach or intestines, is particularly easy. According to the National Institutes of Health, there were about 15,000 gastric surgeries performed per year in the early 1990s, and by 2008 it was in the neighborhood of 200,000.

We know these surgeries are extremely effective in the short term. On the other hand, there are some significant issues in validating success for the long term. First, most studies that have been performed on patients after surgery only followed the subjects for two or three years. Those studies, and rarer studies that follow patients for up to 5 years, do not show a magic bullet for weight loss; but instead show a mixed bag of results and a need for consistent focus and permanent commitment on the part of patients.

Gastric surgeries can vary drastically in complexity from the basic "lap band" – banding a portion of the stomach laparoscopically, to complex re-sectioning which involves remove much of the stomach and substantial portions of the small intestine from the digestive tract, throwing these pieces into a medical waste bin, and re-routing and re-attaching portions of the remaining intestines at new points of insertion.

The *Journal of the American Medical Association* (JAMA) published a survey article that evaluated all acceptable studies of gastric surgery follow-up that had a term of at least 2 years after surgery (Puzziferri, 2014). Several facts are notable, and all of the articles surveyed point to the conclusion that these surgeries are far from a free ride to reaching ideal weight. Unfortunately, the easiest surgeries are the least effective, and the most profound surgeries (involving remove large portions of the digestive tract) are the most effective.

The studies under inspection by JAMA monitored "excess weight loss". Excess weight is weight in excess of "ideal body weight". (Definitions of ideal body weight can vary slightly in studies may have a different methodology than that proposed in Chapter 2, but are all similar – and just like the definition in Chapter 2, represent a target weight based on your height, gender and body composition.)

For the studies considered by JAMA, the average loss of excess body weight is in the 50% range. This means, if you are considering the surgery, that after surgery and two years of a new lifestyle, you can expect to lose on average only half the weight you should ideally lose. You may at this point say "hey, well it takes longer than 2 years".

But wait: There were six studies in the JAMA inspection group that followed patients for a whopping 5 years. Patients in those six studies also had an average "excess body weight loss" of just 49.8%. They had plateaued. Further, the JAMA article suggests that actual statistical outcomes could be worse, because patients who are failing, or regaining weight are more likely to drop out of these studies before they finish than are the successful patients.

Clinicians also report that it is typical after about 2 years for there to be a "creep" effect: after you've lost around half your excess weight, you regain 5 to 15 pounds. This is because your eating habits over time will cause a reduced stomach to re-stretch and grow larger. Reduced intestines in certain surgeries also gain extra efficiency in absorbing food calories. The scariest outcome is that in a fraction of patients, expansion of the stomach pouch continues. This is sometimes called "eating through" your surgery. It happens more or less when patients are taking an "extra bite" of food with every meal for years after surgery, until they "regrow" a large stomach.

There are really no good statistics on how many patients completely relapse from their surgery, especially after 5 years. There has been a mini media circus around certain cases, such as singer Carnie Wilson, who had surgery in the late 90's at over 300 pounds, saw her weight yo-yo over the ensuing years, and finally after losing most of her progress, had a second surgery around 2011. These high profile cases show just how scary and focus-requiring this type of surgery can really be.

Here's what we can conclude about gastric surgery if you look at what long-term data is known and available, and also consider what we've learned so far here:

- These surgeries can be extremely effective to cause very substantial weight loss. If you are determined, you can lose 50- to 70% of your excess body weight within 2 years.

- After about 2 years statistically, you are likely to reach a plateau.

- If you don't make a permanent commitment to eating the correct amount of food and instead view surgery as a magic bullet, not only will your weight loss plateau, you have a decent chancing of eating your way back to obesity.

- If you are 100 pounds or more above your ideal weight, you can count on surgery to help you lose 50 to 70% of this weight in about 2 years. ***If you make the same commitment but avoid surgery, the path to the same weight might take 3 years.*** That's correct, if you adopt the lifestyle you need with surgery, adding on the surgery itself may only save you 12 months.

Relative to the last bullet, really the decision around surgery comes down to the decision to take the surgical risk and to subject yourself to very significant alteration and removal of your digestive tract (for the most effective surgeries), in order to buy yourself some speed.

On the most effective surgery which involve removing portions of your digestive tract, you have to ask yourself the question, "What if I need that later?" If you have a subsequent cancer in the digestive tract, or certain other digestive diseases, your doctor's options in treating these conditions will be significantly more limited after such surgery. If you do justify the surgery, it will certainly be on the basis that the immediate threats to your health from obesity justify those risks.

There are some articles and commentaries in support of gastric surgery that suggest that extremely obese persons have a special disease around obesity that make them singularly susceptible to hunger, and also operate in a metabolic state after weight loss akin to a lower resting metabolic rate. These people are cursed by an underactive metabolism, and will always be able to eat less food than someone who was never fat. Other commentary makes the assertion that once you start losing weight without surgery, your body senses starvation and responds by trying to store more fat.

This type of commentary is comprehensively unpersuasive and nowhere supported by convincing science in my view. We are all different, and some of us are different in the way we deal with impulse control, which is something we'll discuss in Chapter 8; however, the argument that obese persons have some kind of systematic and ongoing handicap is a rationalization to justify surgery that will not permanently untether these patients from the need to learn to deal with hunger anyway.

Only one variable impacts how heavy you get: how much you put in your face. Only one thing drives us to eat too much – excess hunger or perceived hunger. This is an impactor all of us are forced to confront. There are many drivers that impact our level of hunger over hours, days, and weeks, but we know that everyone confronts it at some level, and it must be confronted every day.

If you believe you have a "slow metabolism", exercise is something that is shown to increase it. If your resting metabolic rate is 1,500 calories per day instead of 1,700 calories a day (equivalent to a candy bar) does that justify a rationalization for surgery? Hundreds of thousands (maybe millions) have enjoyed extreme weight loss without surgery – including thousands of persons in the *National Weight Control Registry* discussed in Chapter 8.

For people who are extremely overweight, special pseudo-scientific rationalizations put you into a self-realized victim status. If you start to identify yourself as a victim, you end up being a passive patient, seeking help from drugs and surgery. Because weight loss   with or without extensive medical intervention   requires a comprehensive motivation, focus, and lifestyle commitment. Persons who succeed with surgery do it because they adopt this outlook. Any set of facts or rationalizations that enable you to put yourself in a victim status will nearly ensure your that you fail.

If extra speed is important to you, ***nothing wrong with that***. If surgery is the catalyst that motivates you to do what you need to do, *ok*. It's equally important for you to understand that if you decide to go a surgery route, you are buying yourself some speed and focus, but not a change in the permanent commitment you need to make to eating the correct amount of food.

Why am I always Hungry? Doesn't That Mean I Need to Eat?

This discussion is about hunger, yet we haven't spoken much about beating hunger yet. When it comes to hunger, our body commits the ultimate betrayal. Modern humans evolved mostly during a period between 200,000 years ago, starting in Africa, and 50,000 years ago, when we arrived in Europe. During this period, diet and nutrition evolved, there were numerous periods of climate change, and food was not consistently available. We are omnivores, and while our diets varied to include meat and plant-based food at various times and climatic conditions, all types of food sources we've used are susceptible to short term and long-term variability, due to changes in climate, geography, and seasonal variations.

As a result, our bodies are uniquely adapted to deal with periods of feast, and famine. Unfortunately, one of the "symptoms" of this adaptation is hunger. Our bodies will constantly remind us to eat, and this constant reminder, which we commonly call "hunger", is a naturally selected trait that optimizes survival in a universe of variable food. Early man (and woman) had no reliable means to store food outside the body – no refrigeration, no protectable storage silos, and overall difficulty in amassing surplus. If our body would constantly remind us to eat, it increased the chance that we would eat a lot of food whenever it would be available, and then store it internally.

The biological diseases that are the impact of excess food are not health impacts that we could rely on evolution to correct: these diseases (diabetes, heart disease, and stroke) are either "old person" diseases, or diseases caused by such a gross surfeit of raw sugar and food that they would have been unheard of during most of our evolutionary history. As you may be aware, evolution does little to select away diseases and maladies that appear after the reproductive years.

Fortunately, today is different. We live in a constant river of food. Food is continuously available and actually in such surplus, that we throw about 30% of our food right in the garbage according to some estimates (McGinty, The Difficulty in Taking a Bite out of Food Waste, 2015). Food is a recreation that drives a large sector of the global economy. Businesses that sell food don't want you to eat less – they have to explain to shareholders why they didn't sell 5% more food every year. Restaurant corporations have the same objective. Unfortunately, you are the repository for this sales and marketing effort, and your digestive tract is the victim of this over-aggressive allocation of social resources. You may as well just put your mouth up to the end of a virtual grocery conveyor, which the great economic engine of a global food industry aims to drive a little more and a little faster every year.

(Our aim is not to trash the food industry, which also endeavors to increase sales with more innovation, better products than competitors, and finding new markets. It's only to put your habits in context with our environment, and to remind you that they will gladly sell you more food if you'll buy it. It's your job to figure out how much to eat, not the job of Nestle, Kraft, or Nabisco.)

When you look at the current biological context of food availability, relative to our 200,000 year evolutionary history, you can understand that the last ~125 years represent an unusual blip in availability of food in "First World" societies.

Evolutionary History *of 200,000 years -> food supply variable, eating for survival*

<<versus>>

Modern History *of 125 years -> food supply infinite, eating for entertainment*

It is for this reason that the endocrinological mechanism we call "hunger" is completely, totally, and comprehensively un-anchored from what we need to eat in the modern age. Hunger is really an artifact of conditions that existed during a long period of human evolution. It's for this reason that every person who has a desire or motivation to maintain an ideal weight must accept and understand that hunger provides no meaningful signal about when we should eat, how we should eat, or the correct amount of food to eat. It also means that in order to reach an ideal weight, **we must develop strategies that empower us to disregard hunger**.

In the absence of such strategies, for many of us "coping" means eating intermittently all day as long as we are awake. From an evolutionary perspective, it should be clear that this pattern of continuous eating is not natural. It is also not healthy. Keeping your metabolic system continuously a digestion mode is like taking the air conditioning in your house down to 62°F and letting it run like that without pause. Eventually the equipment will wear out. In the same vein, driving your metabolism with a ceaseless river of food has numerous impacts on health and longevity which we've discussed and will re-visit when I address fasting in Chapter 5.

Constant eating keeps your body in a metabolic state that makes it very difficult for you to burn fat. I spoke earlier about the need to create a calorie deficit of about 500 calories per day to lose a pound per week. This is roughly equivalent to a Snickers bar and a glass of sweet tea.

When you are *close in your consumption of calories to your expenditure of calories*, your body will constantly nag you for a "little bit more food". This is a battle most people lose on most days. You may make it through dinner with that 500 calorie deficit. But you are so damn hungry, and you are watching *House of Cards* at 10PM, and you decide you just won't make it until bedtime. So you have some popcorn with parmesan cheese, a piece of turkey, and a glass of water. BANG! That was the last 500 calories. No weight lost today. Without creating a meaningful prolonged deficit of calories, it is nearly impossible to force your body into the "ketonic" state it enters when you are burning fat.

A CASE STUDY ON JANE'S MIS-ADVENTUROUS WEEK OF DIETING

Jane is a real personal training client of a friend of mine. She has all the basic ingredients to lose weight: exercise, conscientiousness about diet, and acceptance that she needs to change habits:

"I work out four times a week, I am very conscientious about what I eat, I'm dedicated to my program, and I've accepted the fact that being at the correct weight is a lifestyle not a fix. What is wrong? Why can't I lose weight? All this advice is failing me!"

In order to figure out why Jane hasn't lost weight, Jane is asked to log everything she ate for the week. Her goal is to create a daily deficit of 650 calories – a pace of losing about 5 pounds per month. Her four workouts a week include 1 day playing indoor soccer and three aerobics classes per week. She used the tools in Chapter 3 to calculate that she burns about 2,350 calories per day, so that she could eat 1,700 on average in order to lose 5 pounds a month. We asked Jane to write down everything she ate on the first week. At 650 calories a day, Jane wants a total deficit of 4,550 calories by the end of a week.

→ On **Monday** Jane followed her diet plan and worked out (Mon = -650)
→ On **Tuesday** Jane also followed her diet plan but didn't exercise (Tue = - 100)
→ On **Wednesday** Jane worked out, but had lunch with a coworker of a grilled chicken sandwich with fries and a sweet tea, at over 1,100 calories for lunch alone she ate 500 calories more than she burned (Wed = +500)
→ On **Thursday** Jane worked out and mostly followed her diet plan, but she had nachos and a couple cocktails after work with friends (how often?). This is something she only does once a week, but it adds 1,200 calories to the day. She ended up at 2,850 calories (Thu = +1,150)
→ On **Friday** Jane mostly followed her diet plan. She had some chips and a candy bar in the afternoon, which wasn't intended, so she didn't meet her target calorie balance (Fri = -300)
→ On **Saturday** even though it was the weekend, Jane got focused on catching up. She followed her diet plan (-650 calories) and also did extra cardio (-450 calories) so she had a great day (Sat = -1,050)
→ On **Sunday** Jane took it easy as always. She was sedentary, and also ordered food to the house. She nearly followed her diet plan – and would have burned 600 excess calories, but the sedentary day spent lying down took 500 of those away. (Sun = -100)

When you add up the figures for each day of the week, which Jane perceived as a week of extreme deprivation, you will conclude that at the end of the week, Jane did indeed create a deficit … of 550 calories for the entire week. That's less than her objective for one day. This type of outcome is very common. For this week, she loses about 2.5 ounces – an amount that is barely perceptible. It would take her about a month and a half to lose a single pound. And then for the following week – a single additional donut (which co-workers frequently bring to work), and she'll have no deficit at all. No wonder, despite constant focus and self-deprivation, and time in the gym most days, Jane cannot seem to see herself losing weight. Jane's problem is not that she rewards herself, it's that she doesn't know how to ration her rewards or how to plan them. These are topics we'll discuss in Chapter 5 and Chapter 8.

YOUR HUNGER AND YOUR ACCOUNTABILITY

At this stage of this discussion, it will be inevitable for people to start to consider the fact that some of us may be more "cursed" with the demon of hunger than others. Hunger is an endocrinological phenomenon. It's accurate that the nuances of hunger, hormones, or impulse control are not identical for every person; however, we should not place too much significance in this. Too many of us seek to select ourselves into a handicap to explain bad behavior. This nearly ensures failure. The reality is that each and everyone is addicted to food.

There are a couple of basic truths that apply to all of us struggling with hunger. First, with the exception of certain very rare genetic disorders that can cause continuous hunger, most of us deal with similar cycles of hunger every day. In fact, everyone starts to feel hungry just 2 to 4 hours after a satisfying meal. Moreover, as we age, the demon of hunger becomes more persistent: Hunger increases, and we start to feel hungry more continuously. Some of us have struggled with hunger since childhood. For all of us, as we age, hunger becomes increasingly un-related to our biological needs.

There are a few things going on that drive changes in our patterns of hunger as we age. First, excess food in pre-pubescent and pubescent humans can be diverted to growth by our bodies. This is why there is good evidence that the average height of juveniles is greater today than it was 125 years ago. (Natashalh, 2014; Lazarus, 2012). Despite popular perception, estimates of final height in adults have not changed that much; however, good evidence shows that intermediate heights for juveniles are significantly higher. The fact that adult height shows significantly less increase than juvenile differences, suggests that the excess of food available to adolescents may mean earlier growth. Once you stop growing, whenever that happens, failure to reduce caloric intake starts to make you fat.

There are two key hormones that govern hunger. *Ghrelin* makes us feel hungry and *leptin* makes us feel satisfied. As we age, there is some evidence that that the ability of our hypothalamus to make certain co-factors that process and regulate leptin gradually abates (Sahu, 2003).

As you move to and through adulthood, you are starting to be hit by a triple threat to your ability to deal with the burden of hunger:

- you become less active as you leave the "playing" world and enter the working world,
- you are no longer diverting substantial calories to growth and development,
- you are seeing a gradual reduction in your ability to process hormones that signal satiety (the feeling of fullness and satisfaction)

Ultimately, if you are in the throes of middle age, you may realize you are feeling hungry "all the time" when you are awake. Your body is playing a cruel trick on you. Even if you don't enter adulthood with a weight problem, if you don't know how to deal with hunger, you will gradually gain weight all through the course of middle age.

(Research on aging shows that eventually – maybe by your late 60's or in your 70's – your appetite will abate for other reasons. Unfortunately, by this time, you are as fat as a whale and all the health damage has already been done.)

So let's take a second and summarize what we've established so far:

- While there may be differences between individuals, we all get hungry every day and fairly quickly after eating.
- Hunger is a phenomenon that never goes away for more than a couple hours while we are awake.
- Because hunger is an evolutionary artifact, its incidence has no bearing on the correct amount of food we should eat.
- If we don't have a hunger and weight problem in childhood, we'll still have to confront the challenge through adulthood.
- We're used to suppressing urges around things like sex, or resorting to violence. To be healthy and successful we have to learn to suppress hunger.

So, the sensation of hunger is little-related to our actual need for food. Gosh, nature plays cruel tricks, doesn't it? The amount of times I have the urge to have sex also has nothing to do with the number of children I need. And I don't gratify every urge I have around sex. And I'm doing ok. So I guess I need to apply the same principals of restraint to eating as I apply to fornication.

Here is how we have to think of hunger. ***Hunger is a natural addiction.*** Some of us are addicted to alcohol. Some of us get addicted to drugs. Many of us are addicted to obsessive behaviors like hoarding or biting our nails. *But everyone is addicted to food.* To make matters worse, we need to eat food almost every day, so that makes us like an alcoholic who, instead of conquering disease by abstention, has to take a couple of shots each day and then stop drinking. Is it any wonder that we see populations who are 70% overweight in an environment where food is limitless?

Some of us are addicted to drugs or alcohol. Some are addicted to compulsive behavior. Some are addicted to sex. All of us -- 100% -- are addicted to food.

It's this set of facts that often lead us to conclude "society made me fat". We are constantly regaled by CDC statistics about the "obesity epidemic". It's a societal phenomenon. It's an American phenomenon. It's a fast food phenomenon. I got fat because no one will regulate what is served to me at Wendy's, Burger King, and McDonalds. I got fat because the FDA told me that fat was making me fat and that I should eat less fat. So I ate more carbs. And carbs made me fat.

All of this is bullshit. If you got fat, you got fat because you ate too much. If you had reduced your fat like the FDA plate suggested, and not replaced it with carbs (like the FDA also suggested), you'd be fine. Remember that FDA plate doesn't tell you how much to eat, it tells you how to distribute your foods, and probably incorrectly. Did the FDA tell you to eat too much? Social comparisons between US, and say Europe for example don't teach us anything about why we're fat. They only teach us that in the US, it's more socially acceptable to be fat.

Remember how we discussed in Chapter 1 that your weight would impact your career and social success, and also your romantic and interpersonal success? In certain societies, being obese is not socially acceptable. Being somewhat overweight might be ok. Guess what? Being even "somewhat" overweight is not ok for your health. If you are 30 pounds overweight, it's not OK for your health, even if that seems to be OK in Europe. (By the way, global health statistics show that Europe is starting to catch up to the US on this obesity epidemic.)

When we talk about an obesity epidemic, or a society that pushes food, or parents that overfed us as children, or a genetic proclivity to be fat (if that's what's driving this by the way, why do we have an epidemic in the US, one of the most genetically diverse nations on earth). What we are talking about is a very basic breakdown in personal accountability that, unless corrected by you, will ensure your failure in reaching ideal weight. If you are a fat adult, are your parents still putting that food in your mouth? Usually your doctor will give you some great advice, and maybe even a pill or a surgery. Those won't solve a weight problem. Is your doctor responsible if you stay overweight? If you develop heart disease, who is going to deal with the costs, symptoms and consequences? *You are*. Nobody else will give you those daily insulin shots. You have to do that. Nobody else will get you to the correct weight. You have to do that.

So the bottom line here is *STOP PUTTING YOURSELF IN SOMEONE ELSE'S HANDS*. If you spend money at *MediFast*, great if you enjoy it. But your fatal mistake will be when you are sitting around thinking "I've been told if I follow MediFast, exactly, if I eat these pre-packaged meals, I will lose this weight". Again, bullshit. Only what you put in your face, and how much you burn makes the difference (please go back and look at Figure 5). Later I am going to talk about the value of tight feedback loops (frequent weighing, for example) so you can monitor the consequences of your actions. Frequent feedback is the only way you know if you are becoming successful. Casting about for the perfect plan designed by someone else is the same as your casting about for a "cure" for your hunger. It isn't going to happen.

Lest you think this is a non-prescriptive lecture, and you are ready to throw this book aside, let me assure you this isn't the case. In this chapter, the next chapter, and in Chapter 8, I will provide tools you need to be successful and remind you of the enormous rewards in eating. The points being made here are twofold:

- The tools I provide for dealing with hunger may be by perfect for you, or conversely you may develop your own tools and techniques that enable you to reach the same success in a slightly different way.

- Your future weight is a function of only your current weight, your eating, and your activity. Only you control the last two variables. Unless you take personal accountability for your weight, you have no chance of succeeding in reaching your ideal weight.

So what's the happy news in all of this? Well one thing is that we all have to deal with hunger (misery loves company). We can watch with envy our children who are still growing, and can eat as much as they like. For most of the rest of us, we need to average around 1,500 to 2,500 calories per day. That's pretty hard when we are barraged by at least 10 advertisements per day for delicious burgers at quick-service restaurants that can contain 1,000 calories alone. But guess what, we are all in this together, and even when we consume calories in balance, there are many rewards in food.

THE END-GAME OF HUNGER

Here's a great reason for you to confront and conquer the challenge of getting comfortable with hunger. It should be well established at this point that adults – especially getting into middle age – who eat fully as many calories as they burn are still going to feel hungry often. Said another way, even if you eat the correct calories to maintain your weight, you'll still feel hungry often.

...even if you eat the correct calories maintain your weight, you'll still feel hungry often.

If you aren't eating with a perfect energy balance of *Calories eaten = Calories burned* (Figure 5), you will either gain weight or you will lose weight. If you eat more than you burn, you will gain weight.   If you burn more than you eat, you will lose weight. Suppose you have eaten more than you have burned for ten years. You got fatter and fatter, and became less and less active. Suppose you reached 475 pounds which is 290 pounds over your ideal weight. At that point, your weight became so debilitating that you decided to try to lose weight. Now suppose you've been stuck at 475 pounds for the past 3 years.

Well guess what? You are not gaining any weight. That means you are in overall balance and eating the same number of calories you burn. So at 475 pounds, you are experience exactly what you would experience as a healthy person at an ideal weight. The joy and ability to eat, say 2,400 calories per day and stay in balance. Unfortunately you are doing it from a state of miserable conditions of health and well-being. If you are going to "suffer with balance", wouldn't it make more sense to do it at ideal weight?

My point is that for 99.99% of the people who are overweight will eventually get to a weight that is intolerable, at which point we reduce calories and stop continuously gaining weight. So we've already solved half the puzzle: **how to maintain a certain weight**. Now we only have to learn the other half – **how to reach our ideal weight**. Once we get there, many of us will enjoy the same balance of food we were eating before or diet.

The fact is that nobody can keep gaining weight forever, unless they eventually kill themselves (that's the other 0.01% of the overweight). So at some point you must reach that balance. If you are overweight, it only makes eminent sense to swallow hard, calculate your ideal weight, calculate your allowed daily calories to reach that weight, and then enjoy normal eating at the correct weight.

COPING WITH HUNGER

So how do we cope with hunger? When you read the next chapter on fasting, you'll begin to realize that a major weapon in coping with hunger is understanding it. What's the longest waking period you've been without food in the past ten years? For many of us who are overweight, it's been a long time since we went more than a couple of waking hours, if ever! Understanding the mechanisms of hunger, how it affects you, how you react, and learning that it is not the scary intimidating monster you've always concluded is a major part of the evolution of learning and coping.

While fasting will help you to learn the nature and the extent of the hunger beast, there are days when you will be hungry when you are not in a comprehensive fast. It could be a low-calorie day or just a point in time when you've eaten all you should for the day.

This is a good place to start to introduce some of the strategies that will help you cope.

Here are five key *functional responses* that should get you thinking about what you can and have done to address temporal feelings of hunger:

> *Redirect your Energy* – exercise, cook (yes, cooking for other people or for later consumptions is a great diversion), if you've been inside, attack a project outdoors, if you've been sitting, vacuum or laundry, if you've been active, engage your mind

> *Change Your Environment* – very closely related to the last one, if you've been in your office, walk around and connect on important work issues with peers or employees, do a project outdoors, go to the gym or hit a treadmill in your house, run your errands

> *Bait and Switch* – have broccoli or carrots easily available, instead of candy, put healthy food in your office, pre-portion your food before you go to work, eat frequent small planned meals, use caffeine (stimulants are great in moderation), have nuts available (great hunger busters), think about the next reward (restaurant, donut day, whatever)

> *Change your Patterns* – always eat in the morning even if you're not hungry? Skip breakfast for a few days. Always eat out for lunch at work? Trying bringing a sack of food to eat throughout the day. Always have three square meals? Try five small ones. Eat extremely small calories on some days, and more on other days

> *Wait* – Most people think eating is the only cure for hunger because they don't wait long enough. Even if you are very hungry, if you wait long enough, you will learn that your hunger goes away.

> *Tweak Your Diet* – Much discussion, and hundreds of diet books are predicated on the assertion that you will feel less hungry with certain diets. At the end of the day, if you want to reach your ideal weight, you'll have to deal

with some hunger. That being said, there is one dietary pattern that will give you an extra dose of hunger: when you eat a carbo bomb, your body overproduces insulin to soak it up, your blood sugar drops, and you get a rebound hunger. You can reduce some of this treachery by eating few carbs, and using carbs with lots of fiber. Other than that, diets that tell you they'll cure hunger are to a fault, bullshit. Here are some other things you can do around eating to help you deal with hunger, none of it a "cure": 1—drink water when you feel hungry: sometimes you think you're hungry because you're dehydrated, and water uses room in your stomach; 2 – eat foods with a lot of in-digestible fiber (vegetables, whole grains). Takes up room in your stomach and causes your food to be digested over time; 3 – eat slowly so your stomach has time to tell your brain its full (I have trouble with this one). 4 – Eat more protein. This is the inverse of the carbo-bomb diet. Much research has shown better reported satiety after eating high protein meals than eating a carbo-rich diet.

Enjoy Hunger and Enjoy Food *– Maybe you've seen that t-shirt that says "Sweat is your fat melting". You are now wearing a virtual shirt that says, "Hunger is my fat melting". Think about your hunger and know that if you eating the correct amount of food, that hunger is your fat disintegrating. On this basis, with practice, you'll learn to enjoy and appreciate that sensation. For your oral fixation, find small rewards – caffeine is both a reward and an appetite suppressant. Drink a flavored water. Savor it. Reward yourself. Eat a donut, eat at McDonalds, eat at a restaurant and eat what you want. If you are eating the correct calories over the course of days and weeks you can and should do this. When food is a reward instead of a constant assault, you'll enjoy it more and feel more rewarded.*

I realize you may find some of this condescending. Or you are immediately starting to make your brain refute it. "I have to work, I can't just leave to 'change my environment'", etc. etc. Let's put this in context. The themes are more important than the examples. Rather than saying "this won't work for me," I need you to challenge yourself to think of three more tactics for each of the five functional responses above that could be relevant for you. For example "Tweak Your Diet" -> "I could pack lunches for work with no refined carbohydrates". Please stop reading and do this right now. Use the pages at the end of this chapter.

EXERCISE PREVIEW: LIST THREE SPECIFIC THINGS READER COULD DO AROUND REDIRECT ENERGY, CHANGE ENVIRONMENT, BAIT AND SWITCH (CONTROL WHAT IS EASILY AVAILABLE), CHANGE PATTERNS (WHEN YOU NORMALLY EAT), TWEAK YOUR DIET (WHAT YOU EAT). (EXERCISES AND THOUGHT PROVOKERS ARE AT THE END OF THE CHAPTER.)

You may also wonder why I barely included here a category on diet-driven hunger reduction, other than the bullet above "Tweak Your Diet".   You will hear people say that, "If I eat "X", I'm not hungry for a long time, or if I eat "Y" I feel more satisfied. While it is true that managing carbs can help reduce rebound hunger, \that's about all you have to learn in this specialty. Hundreds of diet books that tell you how to eat and not feel hungry are simply selling you the fantasy that you can diet without hunger.

Most of us think "eating" is the only cure for hunger.   There is another: waiting. Hunger always goes away.

The examples should get your determination juices flowing. You may have noticed that not all of the tactics are wholly consistent. Should I eat many small meals or skip meals? Well, fuck, what helps you get through the day? A lot of people swear by many small meals. Other says it brings them into continuous temptation. Some people do better by skipping meals. That takes food off the table. Do what works for you, or do both on different days. That keeps it interesting and keeps you on your toes. The important things are that you create change that belays your focus on hunger – change your environment, change your focus, change your context.

> **EXERCISE PREVIEW**: WHAT DID YOU TRY? HOW WELL DID IT WORK FOR YOU? REMEMBER, REDUCING HUNGER IS NOT THE GOAL, REDUCING EATING IS THE GOAL — SO IF YOU WERE HUNGRY, BUT STILL MANAGED YOUR DIET, YOU SUCCEEDED.

These types of redirects are used by everyone who successfully controls appetite. Think about accountability: You can't eat every time you are hungry, so you must shift your frame and focus. You have to figure out what works for you.

Most people make the mistake of assuming that *the only end to hunger is eating*. That is not actually true. Have you ever gone to bed hungry, and then you wake up early the next morning and maybe you aren't so hungry for an hour or so after you get up? Well shit, it's been nine hours! The reality is that in the short term, your body goes through different hormonal and metabolic states that cause your sensations of hunger to change, even if you are not eating.

The *five functional responses listed* above are about change. If you learn the right strategies to change your focus, change your environment, change your food context, or change your habits, after a time, your hunger will go away. It may not go away for a couple of hours, and it will come back, but it is this type of variability that gets you through your day.

SUMMARY OF WHAT WE'VE LEARNED

Here's what we should have learned and discussed in this chapter.

1. In order to lose weight you have to be hungry. Drugs or surgery can help reduce the time and intensity of feeling hungry, if you decide to invest the money, take the risks, and tolerate the side effects. But no approach, including drugs or surgery, will banish hunger if your aim to reach and maintain your ideal weight.

2. In order to win this battle, you need to learn what it feels like to be hungry and then teach yourself to conquer it. Hunger has no more to do with the correct amount of food than your sexual appetite has to do with your required amount of sex. Understand how to be comfortable with the correct amount of food, and then learn to conquer hunger. You want to lose weight. How do you lose weight? By being hungry. Your hunger is your fat melting.

There are many diet plans and programs that profess to help you "cure" hunger. Diets and programs that promise a cure to hunger are often misleading or worse. For example, programs that talk about eating many small meals per day: This theory is that constant eating keeps you fueled and keeps appetites more level. It can be worthwhile for athletes or fitness fans who exercise often. However, it requires a great deal of discipline. Like telling an alcoholic, "Just make sure you always have a beer in your hand." If you are losing weight, frequent small meals don't banish hunger, and they expose you to the risk of required meticulous portion control. Since small meals don't satisfy hunger, it's possible that you could actually eat more.

The practice of eating many small meals throughout the day has nevertheless captured public consciousness and is widely believed as a healthy practice. A 2015 report from the market research firm Mintel suggested that many snackers believe it's healthier to eat snacks throughout the day rather than big meals. But research, while limited, has not backed it up. A study in the journal *Obesity* concluded that obese men given either 3 meals or 6 meals reported no difference in daily hunger or desire to eat. Another small study of subjects with Type 2 diabetes published in *Diabetologia* concluded that subjects eating only breakfast and lunch lost more weight and had better management of blood sugar than those eating six meal of the same total calories (Consumer Reports, 2015).

The idea that certain diets (beyond the simple "tweaks" mentioned above) don't cure overall hunger should be liberating. No more time to waste trying and rejecting plans that didn't "work" by curing hunger. Now you're ready to confront hunger on your terms. If you eat fewer calories than you burn, you will spend time feeling hunger.

For some people, diet plans and aids will help you with that confrontation. If you think it helps – great – use it with the right expectations.

I have spoken in this chapter about the frame-changing functional responses that can help you to pivot when you feel that hungry. What you will understand by the end of the next chapter is that *fasting* is actually one of the best ways of dealing with hunger. While this may sound counterintuitive, the fact is that while you are in a mode of continuously eating, and continuously fueling your energy requirements with blood sugar, you are also on a continuous cycle of eating and feeling hungry a few hours later. When you fast, your body will feel hungry for the few waking hours, and then you are effectively in a different non-hungry zone.

In the next Chapter, I will discuss fasting and its benefits in driving your body to fat-burrning states, its impact on weight loss, how it teaches you to feel comfortable with hunger, and the many healthy and performance benefits that come from fasting. Then, after a brief discussions on exercise and nutrition, I am going to deliver to you some practical plans and patterns to help you live a life that drives you to your ideal weight.

Exercises – Chapter 4 *Hunger*

Completing these exercises will help you understand your own relationship with hunger.

1. List a few commercial methods of dieting you've tried (shakes, books, groups, etc.). Describe one or two things you've tried on your own.

1	
2	
3	
4	
5	

2. What diet methods (commercial or personal) do you feel were helpful or enjoyable?

1	
2	
3	

3. What methods do you use (or plan to try) to deal with hunger? Label them from the list of functional responses in the chapter (change your environment, tweak your diet, etc.).

1	
2	
3	
4	

4. What hunger coping methods did you try this week? Did they work? (May take more than one week for coping method to work!)

1	
2	

5. Have you considered interventions to deal with hunger (drugs, surgery)? What
is your current view?

1	
2	

Chapter 5 – Fasting

This chapter is organized in two parts. Just as I used the first chapter of this book to sell you on the health benefits of reaching your ideal weight, I'm going to use the first couple pages of this chapter to sell you on the health and wellness benefits of fasting. After that, we'll discuss **why** and **how** to use fasting in the process you will use to reach and maintain your ideal weight.

There has been a tremendous increase in the understanding and meaning of research around the impacts of fasting in the past few years. The benefits of fasting are so comprehensively manifest, worthwhile, and important, that it pays for you to realize and appreciate their impact, beyond the simple benefits of weight management and control. Many people fast for health reasons having nothing to do with weight. That being said, in addition to potential health benefits, intermittent fasting can give you a huge boost in reaching your ideal weight.

THE BENEFITS OF FASTING

I touched on some of the evolutionary support for the natural cycle of fasting in our discussion on hunger. For almost every higher animal, when you look at our biological history, the supply of food is inconsistent and variable. For humans, modern evolution spans about 200,000 years, but food has only been consistently available for many populations for 100 years (and for many, still is not consistently available). Our bodies are adapted to variable food. A bear's health is connected to the cycle of hibernation, and the human body is not as healthy when it is assaulted with food constantly, without the ability to rest and cycle the metabolism.

Eating continuously while waking – as an activity, out of sheer boredom, while watching TV – is like running a car engine at a continuous redline, and never having that vehicle serviced. Your metabolism, your organs, are worn out, exhausted, with no meaningful time for repair or recovery.

In a natural environment with variable food, your body will first signal hunger as supplies of the energy-carrying sugar **glucose** begin to get low. As this process starts, your body starts to use the hormone **glucagon** to signal your liver to convert stored **glycogen** into **glucose** for ready energy. When all the glycogen is used, which happens over the course of a couple of hours when fasting, your body will enter a state of *ketosis*. In ketosis, metabolic products of fat enter your bloodstream and serve as cellular fuel. You are literally burning fat.

You can't get to burning fat without climbing over a hill of hunger.

Because few of us in first-world societies experiment with fasting, few of us are aware of the impact it has on our health and sense of well-being, both in the short-term and in the long-term. We associate fasting with hunger, possibly certain religious practices, and nothing else.

For your health, there are a number of areas where research has started to illuminate the benefits of fasting. New research has taken fasting out of the balkanized disciplines of asceticism and insular religions.

Researchers of fasting and longevity have made a key observations about the health benefits of fasting related to its impact on the level of a hormone I have not yet discussed: **IGF-1** (insulin-like growth factor-1). Persons who eat continuously (most of us) seem to have levels of this hormone that are unnaturally high. It appears that high levels of this hormone may contribute to heart disease, cancer, cardiovascular disease, and age-related ailments.

Valter Longo of the USC Longevity institute has done a great deal of research on this topic (Wade, 2011). In conjunction with his research, he has studied a population of persons in remote villages in Ecuador with a rare genetic mutation called *Laron Syndrome*. These individuals have very low production of IGF-1, which results in low growth during puberty and very small size in adults. The individuals with this mutation have been observed to have zero incidence of cancer, diabetes, and heart disease, despite frequently unhealthy lifestyles including smoking and obesity. You read this correctly: zero. Researches have not identified a case of cancer or heart disease among Laron-bearing population.

Dr. Longo has also suppressed IGF-1 in mice, finding that these mice, like the Ecuadorians with Laron syndrome, live 30- to 40% longer. This would be equivalent to an additional 30 years in human life span. Roundworms modified to suppress IGF-1 have double the normal lifespan (Valter D. Longo, 2003). IGF-1 causes cell division and growth. It's very important to children in puberty, but for adults it contributes to aging.

While the science in this area is incomplete, Dr. Longo believes that during fasting, very significant reductions of the levels of IGF-1 in the blood allows the body to enter a recovery mode, during which cell damage and oxidation are repaired.

Cellular repair includes destruction and disposal of old or malfunctioning cells and destruction and disposal of old or broken proteins (usually enzymes). This process of identification and destruction is driven by small cellular organs called **lysosomes** and the process is called **autophagy**. Autophagy is a critical clean-up process that gets rid of waste, improves metabolic function, and is believed to prevent diseases and disease states, including cancer (which can be caused by failure to identify and destroy old or malfunctioning cells) and heart disease. Furthermore, defects in the process of autophagy are a common denominator in both Alzheimer's and Parkinson's disease (Moussa, 2016).

When you swim in an ocean of forward metabolism, cells do not have time or mechanisms for repair and are more likely to exhibit cancer-causing mutations or inflammatory disease. Studies have shown that short term fasting "upregulates" (i.e. increases) autophagy in many organs including the liver and brain (M Alirezaei, 2010).

Because few of us experiment with fasting, few of us have the opportunity to experience the impact it has on our personal health and sense of well-being, both in the short-term and in the long-term. The need to enter ketosis to burn fat, and the better understanding of the role of IGF-1 in aging have sparked great recent interest in this topic. In fact, much of the change in views on fasting has come in the past 5 years. We are not yet in the mainstream, but at the beginning of a revolution in thinking about natural patterns of food and eating.

For long term health, the following are observed benefits of intermittent fasting:

>**Longevity** – A family of benefits possibly driven by the potential of fasting to mediate of levels of IGF-1, excite autophagy, and enable cellular repair. In certain animal studies, fasting increases life expectancy by 30- to 40% (mice). Suppression of IGF-1 can increase life expectancy from 40% (mice) to 100% (roundworms). These are animal studies. All caveats apply.

>**Prevention of Cognitive Decline (Parkinsons, Alzheimers)** – Studies conducted by the *National Institute of Aging* showed that mice fed every other day

were able to fend off neurotoxins that damaged brain function in ordinary mice. It is believed that fasting increases production of neurotropic factors that are critical for brain development, learning, and memory (Martin B, 2006).

Reaching Ideal Weight – Krista Varady, nutritionist at the University of Chicago researching weight loss concluded that persons can lose weight with a fasting regime significantly more quickly than with daily calorie restriction. I will discuss the reasons for this later in this chapter. A much more technical observation made in a *National Institute of Aging Report* suggests that intermittent fasting reduces levels of circulating insulin. Lower insulin means that sugar in your blood steam is more readily available for energy needs, and less likely to be embargoed by fat cells. Lower circulating insulin can thus support weight loss (once your body turns sugar to fat, you're on track to be hungry again). Finally, subjects who are fasting show lower levels of Cortisol, the stress hormone that encourages storage of fat (Martin B, 2006).

Better muscle mass and lower cholesterol – according to studies performed on mice at the Salk Institute for Biological Studies in La Jolla, California, mice exposed to periodic fasting had better muscle mass and lower serum cholesterol (Amandine Chaix, 2014).

Diabetes Prevention – Lower propensity to develop Type II diabetes may be due to IGF-1 mitigation, and may be due to lower overall levels of insulin and glucose, driven by intermittent fasting. Eating constantly throughout the day does not enable the body to turn off glucose processing which leads to higher blood sugar, according to Dr. Amandine Chaix at the Salk Institute (Amandine Chaix, 2014).

Prevention of Stroke – Based on a mouse study performed by Mark Mattson at the *National Institutes of Aging*, mice introduced to intermittent fasting had lower levels of stroke (Mattson MP, 2005).

Brain Function, Concentration, Mental Acuity, and Memory – When food is less available, according to research at the *National Institute of Aging*, your brain increases production of *brain-derived neurotrophic factor* (BNDF). This chemical encourages the repair of brain cells and the growth of new brain cells. It leads to improved neuroplasticity (the ability for you to learn new concepts, methods, means of concentrating, and means of performing tasks). Neuroplasticity is prevalent in children who learn new languages, skills, and sports easily, but it is weaker in adults. Intuitively, hunger calls on your brain to work harder and more creatively to find new sources of food.

Studies in this area have shown that rodents who are fasting and hungry perform better on mazes. Would you do your best Sudoku puzzle after a thanksgiving meal? Finally, according to a *National Institute of Aging* scientist, fasting supports higher levels of ghrelin (the hunger hormone). People who are overweight have less of this hormone, which encourages growth of new brain cells, especially in the hippocampus, where memories form. For reasons not understood, persons in their 40's and 50's seem to see an increased impact of reduced ghrelin, which can start you on the path of being seriously old, stupid, and forgetful (David Zinczenko, 2013). Nobel prize-

Energy and Well Being – As I mentioned above, fasting reduces levels of circulating insulin in your bloodstream, so that glucose (your blood sugar) is more easily recruited for effort. This may be one of the reasons those who fast feel more energetic. Subjects also often report a sense of euphoria and well-being that develops over time from intermittent fasting. This may be related to some of the brain benefits of fasting also discussed above.

General Reduction in Inflammatory-Driven Illnesses – there is some discussion in scientific literature that fasting may reduce the severity of a host of environmental and inflammatory issues and diseases including asthma, allergies, insulin resistance, susceptibility to infectious disease, sinusitis, gum disease, arthritis, multiple sclerosis, heart disease, cancer, diabetes. These are all diseases caused are exacerbated by the body's natural inflammatory response. The hypothesis is that fasting allows your body to go into the clean-up and recovery mode we've discussed, supporting not only genetic repair, but enabling cells to purge free-radicals, spent enzymes, and other metabolic waste products. Just like your muscles must recover from strength training in order to grow, metabolic cells need full recovery of the waste products created by eating and food. Much research on these mechanisms remains; however if you have any type of chronic inflammatory ailment, it may be worth evaluating the impact of fasting on your symptoms (Peart, 2015).

Short term impacts of fasting are also increasingly well documented via experience and research.

Energy – Fasting subjects often report increased energy after a certain threshold of fasting. This is generally not immediate but may occur after 6 to 8 waking hours of fasting.

Mental Acuity and Focus – fasting imposes a mild stress on cells which is believed to have an impact on brain function and mental acuity according to

Mark Mattson of the Cellular and Molecular Neurosciences Section at the National Institutes of Aging.

Euphoria and Well-Being – Coupled with increased energy and mental acuity, many fasters have reported a euphoric and sense of well-being, akin to a positive caffeine buzz.

It's important to note that not all short-term impacts of fasting are positive, especially for those who are new to fasting. **Headaches, irritability**, and **persistent hunger** are often reported. I will discuss this more shortly.

At this point I will move on to two more themes: "why" and "how" to incorporate fasting into a weight-loss program. With respect to this quick and enthusiastic survey of the health benefits of fasting, it's important for me to deliver a couple of obligatory caveats. Animal studies on mice and roundworms for longevity can't be translated to a human conclusion without much more research on humans. Also, while many health benefits of fasting are either perceived, or preliminarily validated in clinical observations, much more research is needed to understand the mechanisms and impacts of fasting on your health. What I can say for nearly 100% certainty are the following:

1. There is enough research and clinical indications of the benefits of fasting to make it worthwhile for you to consider evaluating fasting in your weekly routine and determining whether it makes you feel more energetic and improves your health.

2. While not all science on fasting is concluded, the impact of obesity on your health is very well understood and conclusory. If fasting will help you lose excess weight, the benefit of fasting for your health is manifest and unambiguous.

The conventional historical wisdom is that fasting is a dangerous method for weight loss, or somehow linked to eating disorders. I have never seen persuasive evidence of this. In fact, considering our bodies are evolved for an environment of variable food, there is a reasonable argument to say that never fasting is unhealthy. Saying that fasting is dangerous because it is tantamount to starvation – even in our world of infinite food – is akin to saying that swimming is dangerous because when we are underwater for moments, it is tantamount to drowning.

Fad diet books that say "fasting causes your body to go into starvation mode, and work harder to store fat" are nonsense, not supported by even clinical observation, and belie the fact that only your calorie balance can create conditions where your body may store fat. The reality is that most of us eat for reasons other than hunger – and never actually experience real hunger because we never stop eating for long enough while waking. Understanding hunger in the context of fasting helps us to address and manage hunger in the rest of our weekly activities.

WHY TO INCORPORATE FASTING IN A PROGRAM FOR REACHING YOUR IDEAL WEIGHT

Constant eating makes it hard to drive your body into ketosis. In Chapter 8 – Putting it All Together, I am going to talk more about establishing routines that ensure you can reach your ideal weight, including elements of fasting; however, it makes sense to discuss now how fasting may fit into a weight-loss or weight-maintenance lifestyle.

Our bodies are adapted to a variable food supply. That's one of the reasons we have the ability to store fat. Our bodies signal us to eat every day, to ensure we will always eat plenty when food is available. As we age, and become less adept at killing or gathering food, our bodies are even more strident in pushing us to eat whenever food happens to be available.

When you eat continuously every day, you are maintaining your body in a metabolic state that makes it difficult for the body to burn fat. You use glucose for energy and your body doesn't enter the fat burning mode called ketosis. Even if you eat a high-protein / low carb diet, your body will eventually turn the protein into amino acids, which if unneeded to build body tissue, will be stripped of nitrogen and used to make glucose, which is either used for energy or turned to fat. Burning proteins for energy is inefficient but it does occur. A similar cycle happens with the consumption of dietary fats. In fact, K.D. Hall, who has done a great deal of principal scientific research on how the various metabolic pathways impact weight gain and weight loss asserts that your dietary mix (fat / protein / carbs) has little impact on weight loss (Kevin D Hall, 2011), despite hundreds of diet books to the contrary. The key point is that it is difficult to send your body into a state of ketosis (fat burning) if you are eating anything, even if you emphasize protein or fat over carbohydrates.

A slight energy imbalance is hard to manage. One key reason why fasting is important in a weight loss program is that a slight energy imbalance is very difficult to navigate and manage. A judicious goal for someone reaching their ideal weight is to seek to lose one pound per week. That works out to a deficit of about 500 calories per day (i.e. you eat 500 fewer calories than you burn).

Unfortunately, a 500 calorie deficit is so close to calorie balance – actually a glass of orange juice and a cup of yogurt away – that operating in this range while dieting is equivalent to trying to thread a needle --- or to introduce the element of danger --- equivalent to trying to walk on the edge of a razor. Worse you may not know exactly where the razor is that you are trying to walk on: recall we said in Chapter 3 that the calculation of allowed calories is an estimate, because your exact resting metabolic rate is unknown, and changes as you lose weight.

This proverbial invisible razor walking has two implications. First, because you are tantalizing your body with food all day, your body is going to use that immediately available food to meet its energy requirements, and as soon as those glucose and glycogen (stored glucose) reserves run low, your body will nag you with hunger. Most people eventually lose this battle. You may be on top of your shit all day, managing food intake perfectly, and then its 10 PM and you're watching "Walking Dead", and you give in to a bowl of popcorn with cheese. There goes your weight loss progress for the entire day. Unless you are that rare adult who goes to bed at 9 PM and then can sleep for 10 or 11 hours (which means you are pretty boring), it's hard to work at this level of precision for the long periods of time needed to lose substantial weight for several reasons.

First, allowed calories from Chapter 3 may have an error of +/- 200- to 400 calories using the estimation methods in this book. Estimating your resting metabolic rate is imprecise, and estimating your activity-driven calorie expenditure is also imprecise: it's based on a range derived from your own subjective evaluation of how active you are (and most people overstate their activity level). Second, tracking the calories of everything you eat can be extremely tedious, demands constant attention, and is also subject to estimation and uncertainty. Finally, if you actually are able to home in on a deficit around 500 calories, your nagging hunger makes it very easy to miss the mark in the last hours of a day.

The daily allowed calories method is great for giving you a sense of how much you can eat every day – say approximately 2,200 calories. That's why I included it as Chapter 3. It gets you in the correct zip code. However, it's imperfect for a scientific determination that your food intake will drive you to weight loss.

Fasting helps deliver insurance that you create a real deficit and enter ketosis. In fact, just fasting one day per week off the top ***reduces your calorie overall weekly calorie intake by around 14%***, and would by itself cause you to lose about 3 pounds per month. People may want to assert that if you fast on Monday, you'll ruin it by gorging on Tuesday. Animal studies have shown this is not the case for mice (David Zinczenko, 2013) and (Varady, 2013). Further clinical studies performed by researcher Krista Varady have born this out for both mice and men.

Fasting will make you comfortable with hunger. Typically the first six hours of a waking fast, you are going to feel consistently, persistently hungry. This is a good thing if you are moving into a program of weight loss. As you gain experience with hunger, the "nagging" element of your sense of hunger will abate. Nothing is as good for training you to feel comfortable with hunger as a determined fast. When you realize that you can execute a 24-hour fast with barely a scratch or scar, this will increase your confidence on any elective lower-calorie days that it's ok to eat smaller meals or go on long stretches of the day without putting something into your face.

HOW TO INCORPORATE FASTING IN A PROGRAM FOR REACHING YOUR IDEAL WEIGHT

We'll talk more about the topic of establishing a weight-loss routine in Chapter 8, "Putting it All Together", but in order to reach your ideal weight, it's important that you have at least one full 24-hour fast per week. This needs to start with your identifying a day that you can fast with meaningful consistency most weeks of the year.

Table 10 shows you several variations on how you can incorporate a weekly fast into your lifestyle. The most basic fast is a literal 24-hour fast – and in that fast, you might eat after 24 hours and one minute. (I don't encourage watching the clock that closely. After you gain experience with fasting, if you have the right attitude, you should feel no sense of emergency to watch a clock and eat the minute you can. If you do have this attitude you will not be successful. Rather you will psyche yourself into thinking you are starving yourself, which is plainly ridiculous outside our distorted cultural norms.)

24 hour fast. One way to proceed is to start your fast at bed-time. Suppose your day of fasting is Friday. Have dinner at 6 PM on Thursday and then eat dinner again at 7 PM on Friday. If you eat late at night, have a 10 PM snack on Thursday, and then break your fast Friday night with your favorite food or at your favorite Friday night establishment. This is kind of like the Jewish Yom Kippur fast of sundown to sundown (I believe the Jews use 25 hours). Make sure you pass a full 24 hours. Pace yourself when you end a fast. You will find that you fill up on a reasonable amount of food.

Full cycle fast. A more enhanced fast involves starting by skipping breakfast and also breaking your fast at breakfast. When you wake up, if you don't eat, you've already been fasting 8 or more hours asleep. Then you don't eat at all for the calendar day and go to bed as normal. Waking up and in this case literally breaking fast with breakfast you are at about 34 hours. A purist might say that this is the only way to go an entire day without eating. In this approach you have a deeper fast, create a deeper deficit, and you are less likely to overeat at breakfast. Example: eat a later dinner Wednesday night. Get up and go to work and don't eat. Get nice rest on Thursday night and resume your normal routine on Friday.

Your experience starting a fast won't vary that much whether you start at bedtime or upon waking: either way you'll feel hungry for most of the morning. Starting after breakfast does mean that you will go to sleep that night having been fasting … but most persons do not find this to be an issue. By bedtime, you are in a full fast and your body is tuned for resilience against hunger.

Those 5:2 Diets. There are also other perfectly successful variations in how you can fast. Many popular diet treatments recommend a 5:2 fast – two days of fasting per week. This is perfectly acceptable. The only issue is that many of these diets call a day of around 500 calories or less a "fasting day". I don't consider a 500 calorie day a fasting day. That's just a diet, and it could abnegate many fasting benefits: discipline, comfort with hunger, full metabolic turnover, and autophagy.

For learning to develop comfort with hunger, you should choose a day not to eat. In fact, on a fasting day, it's much easier to be successful if you eat no food at all, than if you tease yourself with small amounts of food, and prevent your body from entering a hard fat-burning metabolic state. Avoid "pseudo-fasts". I recommend if you use a 5:2 variation, to use the strict 24-hour fast of zero eating, and to try to separate the fasts by a day or two days if you plan to use this approach every week. Doing so, you may be able to increase weight loss from 1-2 pounds per week to 2-3 pounds per week. Example: Eat dinner on Monday night, don't eat Tuesday until a late regular scale dinner. Do the same thing again either Thursday or Friday.

Mode	Description
24-hour Fast	Start in the evening after dinner. Like the Jews, don't eat again til the 25th hour. Use moderation when breaking the fast.
Full-cycle Fast	Start in the evening after dinner, but take the next entire day without food. Don't eat til you wake the next morning (usually 34 hours).
5:2 Fast	Choose two days a week for a 24-hour fast. Can result in more rapid weight loss.
Multi-Day Fast	Find a two-day window to fast, or a 3 day window. Don't fast more than two consecutive days without discussing with a doctor (see sidebar). Not recommended weekly. Great to get you in touch with the discipline of fasting and comfort with hunger.

Table 10 – Variations on the daily fast.

Remember if you normally eat 2,400 calories a day, your fast doesn't remove all the calories you need to lose a pound per week (which is 3,500 calories). You need to focus on having a couple of other modest deficit days.

The question always comes up --- well can I eat **anything** during a fast. Well first, drink a lot of water. When you wake up, drink at least two 8 ounce glasses of water immediately. Next, if you like coffee, have some coffee. It will help you get through the day, especially the morning. Can I put anything in my coffee? Sure, you can include a teaspoon or two of sugar and a splash of milk. That's about 15 calories. This will have almost no impact on your fast. If your coffee is ¾ of a glass of sweetened milk with a splash of coffee or something you bought at Dunkin Donuts with chocolate chips and 400 calories, that is absolutely not a fast and it is actually enough calories to qualify as a meal.

Later in the day, if you feel you want a little bit of sugar or electrolytes, you can drink a splash of Gatorade in your water. Late afternoon 3 or 4 ounces of Gatorade in a sixteen ounce glass of ice water is ok. If you are taking in 250 calories of Gatorade sugar, you are not fasting.

With respect to the **optimal day to fast** – there is no optimal. In order to make sure you get your fast every week, you need to be selfish about your fast and work around it. You need to consider your weekly cycle and routine, whether you have kids, job-related travel, or other requirements. You should pick a day that you feel you can fast consistently every week. For example, if you are expected to take the employees out to lunch every Friday, then Friday is not a good day to pick to fast (unless you can move that lunch to Thursday). If you consistently travel M-W for work, that block is not a good day to pick unless you consistently have a travel day when you are mostly alone and not expected to eat with customers.

> **EXERCISE PREVIEW**: THINK ABOUT YOUR TYPICAL WEEKLY RESPONSIBILITIES, ELIMINATE THOSE THAT WORK LEAST WELL. AND SELECT A GOOD DAY TO FAST. MUST PICK A DAY AND COMMIT — NOT "IT WILL VARY BY WEEK". EVEN IF YOU TRAVEL FOR WORK, YOU CAN USUALLY PULL IT OFF.

If you don't have a consistent day that you can nearly always fast – you will drive yourself crazy each week. Can I do this today? Is this the best day? Could I fit it in Thursday instead? Do I really feel like it today? I'm really super hungry now and maybe I'll feel more like it on Tuesday. You'll drive yourself crazy and you'll talk yourself out of what you need to do. You won't act consistently. It's really much better to make that personal type of commitment: "...On Fridays (Thursdays, Mondays), we Fast". This is a personal commitment you make to yourself, by yourself, and for yourself.

Do not involve others in the drama of your fast. If you talk about your fast while you are fasting, and how hungry you are, you will drive those around you crazy, and also make it more difficult for yourself. Fasting is your thing. It should be fairly personal, private, and introspective. Keep it low key. I like to fast on Friday. There have been occasions on that day that I've had a breakfast meeting and ordered some wheat toast and a coffee. If I handle and crumble the toast during the meeting, the other guy person rarely seems to notice that I didn't actually eat. If it would be obvious that I am not eating, then that's a day I have to pivot and can't fast. Whatever you do, don't make somebody else feel uncomfortable because you aren't eating.

MULTI-DAY FASTS – PART 1

People who enjoy fasting often ask me about the benefits of a multi-day fast. I occasionally enjoy a multi-day fast, but admit that it is often hard to fit-in with busy schedules, and without annoying the wives, kids, and co-workers in some way. There are benefits in driving self-discipline, introspection, and, according to research, significantly reducing IGF-1. These longer fasts are shown to substantially reduce and reset the levels of IGF-1 hormone in your blood. After you've gained fasting experience, you may decide to consider a two-day or even three-day fast. Here are some guidelines for multiple day fasts:

- Discuss with a doctor first if you plan to consider fasting for more than two days;
- If you are diabetic, do not consider multi-day fasting;
- Don't do a multi-day fast every week. Once per quarter is just plenty;
- If you fast for a second or third day, you'll find that those additional days are easier than the first day, because you don't face those six hours of nagging hunger before the body enters ketosis;
- You need to conscientiously maintain fluids (water) during a multi-day fast;
- For safety, and to make sure you maintain electrolytes, sip an 8-ounce bottle of Gatorade, diluted with water, throughout the day;
- Alternatively, on the second and third day, drink a packet of onion soup in hot water in the morning – this will also help you maintain electrolyte balance at only about 30 calories

WHAT TO EXPECT WHEN YOU ARE FASTING (HUNGER AND FASTING)

You can't get to fat burning without climbing over a hill of hunger … Weight loss is found only on the other side.

On a day that you fast, the first six hours – *the morning* – are the hardest. If you start your fast at bedtime, you'll start to get hungry within an hour or two of waking. For a novice faster, this is the hardest part of a fast. Sure, you are going to be hungry all day, but this is the most nagging part of hunger. If you are at work or engaged in any other regular activity, you are going to find that your mind moves to food every five or ten minutes.

How do you drive through this hunger? You should turn to the techniques in Chapter 4. Mainly *redirect your energy*, and also *change your environment* frequently if it's practical. Drink coffee if you do that. If you don't, drink some hot tea. Drink plenty of fluid to trick your body to think its eating. Most of all stay active and engaged. As your fast proceeds through the day, you will find your focus increases and you may have some of your most productive days.

Note that because you are not eating today, you are going to have a couple of extra hours! Did you ever wish there were 26 hours in the day? Today there are. Use the extra time, and schedule a full set of activities and accomplishments. Remember boredom is the enemy of dieters and it's the enemy of your fast. Stay engaged.

As you move into *the afternoon* you'll begin to feel less hungry. Don't get me wrong, you are going to feel hunger all day. Nevertheless, you won't feel the nag of hunger, you won't feel the oral fixation, and you won't constantly catch yourself trying to grab something to put in your mouth. Your body is moving into ketosis and it has found a new energy source by burning fat. You'll probably also start to feel increased alertness and mental acuity, even if you have not had caffeine. This is a great time to feel productive and get a lot done.

Moving into *dinner time* that feeling of mental acuity will persist, but you may also start to have some negative effects of fasting. First, some people around this time report they have headaches. Fasting takes practice, and if you do have **headaches**, know that most people report that the headaches go away after they've gotten used to the routine of fasting. If they persist for you, realize that you are now in the home stretch and have only a few hours left. The other impact that is common is **irritability**. Consistent with the principal that you don't make drama around your fast, if you have this symptom, you need to keep an internal dialogue frequently reminding yourself that your irritability is your fast, not the annoying people around you. Your irritability may- or may not go away with practice, but with practice, you will learn to manage it. When you understand it's the fast, it's easy to ignore. For some people, breathing, relaxation, or turning on some classical music can help you with your irritability.

Many people ask whether they need to reduce their normal activities, skip exercise, or spend the day in general repose while they are fasting. The answer is absolutely not. You will feel more energy and determination during a vigorous fast. If you have good hydration and electrolytes, you'll have no trouble with vigorous exercise or strength training for an hour. Obviously it's not a day to run the ultra-marathon, but neither is it the Jewish day of rest and introspection. Continuing normal activity ensures your body will harvest energy from fat in a ketonic state. Do what you need to do – work, play, exercise – and your body will step up.

Ultimately, what you will find is that after you've been fasting for a few weeks, you'll begin to look forward to your fast, to enjoy your fast, and you'll feel short-changed if for some reason you have to sacrifice your fast. This is a good thing and ensures that you naturally stay on your program.

Dr. Mark Mattson of the *National Institute of Aging* echoed this conclusion based on two small studies he conducted on subjects who tried intermittent fasting: "The only subjects who dropped out dropped out within the first 2 weeks. After 2 to 3 weeks they got to like the diet, mainly because they started losing weight and started feeling better. It doesn't matter which fast a person does. If they can do it and stick to it, they're going to lose weight and their health is going to improve." (David Zinczenko, 2013)

MULTI-DAY FAST – PART 2

I would not recommend a multi-day fast unless you really enjoy fasting and have spoken to a doctor. There are potential benefits in longevity and IGF-1 control, but multi-day fasting is not a necessary element of weight management or control. Make sure you've established a routine of fasting one day a week and are comfortable with it before you consider testing a multi-day fast. I would not recommend a multi-day fast more frequently than every three months.

If you do periodically fast for more than one day, you will find that day two (and day three if you are hard-core) are easier than the first day. It is unusual going to bed not having eaten, but you are in ketosis. When you wake up, you won't have to deal with that crazy six-hour nagging hunger that goes with a transition into ketosis. You will feel hungry, but irritability becomes manageable and you will feel that heightened sense of mental acuity and alertness through the balance of a long fast.

THE FASTING FAD: FASTING AND SOCIETY

In terms of reaching and maintaining an ideal weight, if you've read this far, you've realized that there is only one thing that matters: **how much** you eat. That's why we've equated success in reaching your ideal weight with the challenge of conquering hunger. Thousands of diet programs amount to detailed prescriptions of **what** you should eat or **when** you should eat. All of these types of programs are often just complex gimmicks that claim to reduce time and intensity of hunger, or in some cases distract you from hunger by giving you a set of complex tasks and menus to perform and follow.

If this is the case, why would the technique of fasting be any different? Clearly it is much simpler than some programs, but at its root, it is really just one more approach to dieting that tells you **when** to eat. I think this is a valid criticism of placing too much importance on the need for fasting in reaching your ideal weight. The argument supporting fasting for weight management is this: Sensible weight loss involves creating a deficit of about 500 calories a day. Such a small deficit is narrow, hard to maintain, causes you to exist in a cycle of nagging hunger enabling you to miss the mark on many days, and makes it difficult to ensure that you'll reach the deep calorie deficit that will drive you in to ketosis (fat burning). Do you have to fast to reach your ideal weight? "No." Do I believe it's ridiculously challenging to succeed in sustained weight loss without fasting? "Yes."

If you are inclined to say, "I just don't like fasting", or "I just don't think I can fast," I would only suggest that you try it for ten weeks before you conclude it has no place in your weight management program. Then if you decide it doesn't work, you can make the same statements credibly.

Hundreds of diet fads have come and gone over the past five decades. Is there any reason to think the idea of fasting to lose weight won't suffer the same fate? I believe the answer to this is a resounding "Yes" for the following reasons:

- Most diets tell you exactly what to eat, how much to eat, and when to eat. Fasting is a lifestyle modification that allows persons to reach and maintain an ideal weight, not a prescription;
- It is very hard to create the calorie deficits that cause the body to start burning fat without fasting;
- Variability of food and fasting are integral in human history throughout evolution, and are part of the context and history of nearly all ancient religions for that reason;
- The health and wellness benefits of creating variability of food and fasting are just beginning to be understood over the past decade. Even at the current level

of understanding, the health and longevity benefits are just too great to be ignored or passed on.

Fasting is not a fad.

If fasting is not a fad, what about the diet revolution around the act of fasting, and the inevitable programs, tools, and books that will come out on this topic (like this one)? What should we make of all that?

I do feel that sometimes these books tend to be too prescriptive. They will tell you exactly what to eat. Sometimes they tell you exactly when to eat. They often include recipes and meal plans. They may tell you exactly how to exercise. They may even suggest more exercise than you actually need (or want). Maybe in some cases this information is to fill the white space, and to help sell books. Some of it can be overwhelming.

Most people have trouble staying on a course of antibiotics three times a day for ten days. (Have you ever guiltily found 2 or 3 pills left at the end of 10 days?) Following a detailed, prescriptive program of cooking, eating, quantities, schedules, and exercise forever is much harder. Our aim here is to give you the basic principles around eating and hunger, fasting, nutrition (Chapter 6), and exercise (Chapter 7) that can enable you to easily find a rhythm and achieve a balance that can realistically fit any reasonable lifestyle.

That being said, there are a few mainstream diet books already on the market, in bookstores, and on Amazon that enthusiastically advocate fasting. The obvious question: what is the worth of these books and programs? The answer for a few of these books is "quite good!" They contain great information, and they stress the value and importance of using fasting in achieving your weight management goals. Since I believe these books contain worthwhile information, it is worth mentioning a couple of them and providing a couple of caveats.

One of the popular books is *The 8-Hour Diet* by diet and fitness author David Zinczenko. In this approach Zinczenko prescribes fasting 16 hours each fasting day, and concentrating all of your meals into an 8-hour period. The approach does not require you to have an "8-hour diet" every day. This discipline could be limited to 2 or 3 days a week, although clearly you'll lose weight much more slowly if you only engage 2 days per week. Zinczenko calls breakfast "the most over-rated meal of the day" – and this is the greatest truism in the book.

The biggest concern I have with this beautiful and simple approach to fasting and weight loss is that the book encourages that during your 8-hour period of eating on fasting days, you can eat as much as you want. Mice and animal studies show that mice consistently restricted to food during an 8-hour period won't eat twice as much food as mice who have access to food for sixteen hours per day. This "selling point" element of this approach doesn't automatically translate to human subjects.

I believe food is a reward, and that you have to reward yourself with decadent food regularly to stay motivated while you are losing weight, but the assertion that you can eat what you want, as much as you want for 8 hours would be enabling for many food addicts. Never underestimate the determination of the insatiable and corruptible American appetite for food. Thousands of people every year eat through stomach staplings and laparoscopic bands for gosh sake! And the mice don't really know that their food will get cut off after 8 PM. You do, and you've been told to eat whatever you want until then.

Another great book on diet in fasting is "The Every Other Day Diet" by Krista Varady and Bill Gottlieb. In Dr. Varady's approach, you eat a 500-calorie diet on "Fast Days" and eat you whatever you want, as much as you want on "Feast Days". Dr. Varady has performed a number of clinical studies on these diets and published her findings in clinical journals. While she does not recommend a full 1-day weekly fast as I have, her Fast Days at 500 calories are seriously fast-like day. For many of us, 500 calories is around half of a single meal. (Varady also heartily endorses that breakfast is over-rated and unnecessary.) From her clinical studies, she has concluded that despite the lack of restrictions, patients eat only 110% of their normal caloric intake on Feast Days, are more mindful of what they eat, and eat more fruits and vegetables.

I think this subject behavior is credible in small clinical studies with participants who are mindful of the objectives, but the cover of the book shows a pepperoni pizza, an iced donut with sprinkles, and a double fast-food burger in its cover graphic, representing the Feast Day. I do worry that for the masses, this simple prescription of "eat whatever you want, as much as you want" on "feast days" may be enabling and not effective in an un-monitored environment. All the recent authors including Varady agree that **weight loss = calories-in – calories-out**, just as we discussed in Chapter 3. No set of simple rules can necessarily prevent you from overeating if you unleash yourself for bottomless food eight hours per day, or four days per week.

Ultimately, you need better guidelines to ensure success. I do advocate one full introspective fast per week. That's almost enough to lose a pound a week even if the rest of the week reflects calorie balance. I also recommend that the dieter select a couple other days to create an obvious calorie deficit – maybe eating 1,000 to 2,000 calories for most persons. Don't try to walk on the edge of that razor blade for six days. I advocate learning to live in balance – eating what you need – this is a great tool for the rest of your life – when you've reached your ideal weight and have decide to maintain it forever. You also need to pick great rewards every week – a restaurant meal where you order whatever you want, your favorite fast food foray, your weekly pot-luck at work.

We'll talk more about how to manage this in uncertainty an uncertain world when we get to Chapter 8.

A number of recent books including this one are recommending that you to go long continuous periods without eating or with eating very little. In the course of doing this, these authors are telling you that you need to 1) restrict calories, 2) spend periods of time fasting, and 3) learn to deal with the consequent hunger. Do you see a pattern emerging here? After about 65 years of focus on diet, nutrition, and weight in the US, we are finally starting to see some coherent patterns around the relationship between weight and diet, hunger, fasting, exercise, and nutrition.

Exercises – Chapter 5 Fasting

Completing these exercises will help you prepare you for fasting.

1. What health benefits discussed in the chapter do you recall --- write a few down. Which do you believe are likely true (if any)? Which would you like to realize?

1	
2	
3	
4	
5	

2. What was the longest period of time that you recall going without eating in the past year? Write about it. If it was more than five hours, write down what you recall being difficult about it? How could you deal with those challenges?

1	
2	
3	

3. Think about your typical weekly routine. What days would work least well? And select a good day to fast EVERY week. Pick a day for a commit – not "it will vary by week". Write down the day you picked:

Day	Reason

4. After fasting on your chosen day, write down what you found difficult and how you dealt. (I always find the nagging instinct to eat for the first six hours the most difficult.) Continue for several weeks and then write if and how your perspective has changed or improved.

AFTER ONE DAY

Challenge	How you dealt with it.

AFTER ONE MONTH (OK TO SAY YOU OVERCAME ANY CHALLENGES)

Challenge	How you dealt with it.

Chapter 6 – Nutrition

We've touched on many themes of nutrition throughout the first five chapters of this book. It makes sense to narrowly explain and crystalize a couple of these key themes. Considering the complexity of the topic, I will try to keep it concise. There are a few reasons for this:

- It can be boring;

- Despite what 40 years of diet books have told you, what you eat (carbs vs fat vs protein) has little impact on how much you weigh. How much you eat has all the impact;

- The mixture of foods you eat can have some marginal impact on hunger, and this is the only tenuous theoretical impact it has on weight. We've mentioned carbohydrates in this context, but for the big picture, everyone who decides to reach and maintain an ideal weight will need to learn to conquer hunger. Your dietary mix has only marginal impact on your overall level of hunger;

- *When* you eat is also oft-cited as a way to reduce hunger. Again, you can't substantially mitigate hunger with timing. Any complex schemes around schedule will have only marginal impact on your hunger. The most important driver of daily hunger also happens to be the only driver of weight loss: the calorie deficit you create;

- If you are overweight or obese – the most immediate and imminent threat to your health is your weight. It isn't the gluten, or the fact that there is too much

Omega-6 in your Canola, or that your apples have 1% of EPA limit of pesticides, or that your cereal is not certified organic. It is that you are fat, you are using your digestive track as a garbage disposal, overworking your metabolism and organs, straining and stressing your heart, and driving yourself into a population of persons with a plague of diabetes and cancer. 99.9% of the threat to your health is your weight. Many of these food fads and trends – like organic, pesticide free, gluten free, grass-fed, cage free, non-GMO – have never been shown to impact health outcomes, quantity, or quality of life. Clear links between obesity and diabetes, heart disease, and cancer have all been established. These three villains are among the top killers of both men and women. Solve the problem by reaching your ideal weight. At that point, if you believe you will earn an extra health benefit by paying up for organic foods (which benefit may be less than 0.5% of the benefit you achieved by reaching your ideal weight, and may actually be zero), then by all means pay up for trendy organic produce sold in a store with the fake hardwood floors. Any such health benefit articulated today is usually based on perceived, but not scientifically established, reduction of cancer risk or some other ailment far in the future. All of this marketing around "organic" and "GMO free" is only taking money out of your wallet without delivering a tangible health benefit. If you are theorizing that focusing on food pedigree – origin, means of preparation, or composition – has any positive benefit for your health while you are sitting on your couch 40 pounds overweight, it's the inane equivalent to your casually saying to your spouse, "Hey I changed the battery in the smoke detector this morning," while your house is actually at that current instant on fire. If you think some of these foods taste better, or if you enjoy the stores where they or sold, or if you think that you might be helping small farmers, or that you are helping to improve the treatment of animals, and you have the affluence to afford high-end food choices, then right there you have a reason to invest in these foods. If on the other hand you are buying these foods as part of a weight-loss, or health improvement mentality, you are wasting money, time, and focus.

- With respect to fat, for a number of "dark age" years you heard that foods that were high in fat made you fat. Now that's been dismissed. Calories make you fat. For years you heard that beef, because it is high in saturated fat, contributes to heart disease; however, this isn't currently well-established in the scientific community. Half the fat in beef is the same healthy fat that occurs in olive oil (Campbell, 2015), and it is possible that the saturated fat in beef may actually improve your levels of good cholesterol. The relationship between dietary fat and the cholesterol and triglycerides circulating in your blood is not completely understood. (I don't have an agenda here for or against beef. I'm only making the point that in the past "settled science" around diet and nutrition has proven wrong. While clinical studies have suggested a relationship between saturated fat and health problems, the science isn't understood and the clinical evidence is not entirely consistent.) Overall level of eating and genetics may have as much or more impact on heart health than the composition of the fats that you eat.

In a nutshell, your composition of protein, carbohydrates, fat, (alcohol), has little impact on what you weigh. It's how much of these things you eat that has impact. And ultimately, nothing related to nutrition has anywhere near the impact on your overall health as your weight does. So focus on reaching your ideal weight above all else. When you've arrived there, feel free to tweak and optimize if it makes you feel good.

...when it comes to nutrition, many of us spend a lot of timing thinking about the quality of our food, but for our health, quantity matters more .

Now that this tirade is over, let's acknowledge that there are a couple truisms around your dietary composition that impact health and must be addressed in a survey of nutrition for dieters. **Example 1**: there is one probable unhealthy fat (trans fats). **Example 2**: gluten does create harm for some people. The next few pages tell you key things you need to know about the caloric food actors (carbs, proteins, fats).

Understanding important well established facts will help you understand your body, manage your trajectory to your ideal weight, and avoid pitfalls that may jeopardize your health. If you are not interested in any more detail than that, then just skip to the end of this chapter "A Simple Precis on Nutrition" – here I summarize facts about nutrition that are widely accepted and established over time, and which you can use to simply modify behavior if you are out of line. You don't have to follow a complex and cumbersome diet program to have good nutrition, and you don't need a Ph.D. in nutrition. There's not an ocean to memorize, and it's not that difficult to live healthy, still eating food that is delicious and satisfying.

For purposes of this discussion on nutrition, there are two kinds of nutrients. Macronutrients have calories and are divided into 4 groups: carbohydrates, fats, proteins, and alcohol. Micronutrients have no calories and fall into three groups: vitamins, minerals, and water. Micronutrients are agents or substances that your body needs to conduct the ongoing chemical reactions that represent life.

CARBOHYDRATES

If there is one nutrient that drives more discussion around diet and hunger than any other, it is carbohydrates. That's why I'm tackling it first. You've probably picked this up reading the book so far, but carbohydrates are either simple sugars (such as sucrose (table sugar) or fructose (fruit sugar)), or complex chains of sugars, sometimes called "starches" (potatoes, bread). Whether you are eating simple or complex carbohydrates, all starches are eventually converted to glucose. Eating a 500 calorie baked potato is not ultimately different from eating 500 calories of table sugar. Glucose is available to give you energy, and it can be stored temporarily as glycogen, mainly in the liver, with limitations. Excess glucose goes into long-term storage as fat.

The question that always comes up in discussions about carbohydrates is this: do carbs make you fat? If you've read this far in the book, you know the answer is "NO". Eating too much is what makes you fat. Guess what? It's very easy to eat too much when you eat a lot of carbs.

Here are the reasons: farming and agriculture has evolved to give us carbo-bombs in what we grow (modern hybrid wheat, eating a lot of potatoes), and food processors have piled on by making carbs even easier to mainline (adding refined sugar to many products, formulating baked goods with white flour). We also naturally crave carbohydrates, just like a hummingbird craves sugar.

Carbohydrates are not villainous. You need energy to get through your day. Carbohydrates provide you energy. Your body uses them first for that. Suppose you are already at your ideal weight so that you have no need to burn fat to shed pounds. If you aren't building muscle and tissue, you don't absolutely need a lot of protein and fat either (you do need some for repair, replacement, enzyme production). You could survive on a diet of mostly carbs for energy (plus the required micronutrients vitamins, minerals, and water), and you might be healthy as a horse. If you cut back on carbs, your body has to harvest energy from proteins and fat, which is less straightforward.

The issue is that carbohydrates are very easy to "overdose" on: a delicious, calorie dense food, widely available, that we naturally crave.

Let's talk about what happens when you eat a carbo-bomb: In a nutshell, your blood sugar starts to increase ("spike"), and with some delay, your body reacts by producing the hormone insulin, which directs your cells to soak up the glucose. If you've eaten a carbo-bomb, your body typically over-reacts. It produces too much insulin, and then your blood sugar soon plunges. This has two negative impacts: a feeling of rebound hunger and a feeling of low energy and lethargy. Have you ever heard the old adage that "Whenever I eat Chinese food, I'm hungry an hour later." The basis of that legend in fact might be that the white rice, if overeaten, is creating an insulin response which causes your blood sugar to drop after that rice is metabolized.

Let's talk about what happens to the glucose that comes from your carbo-bomb: Some is taken up by your cells for energy. Some is stored in your muscles and liver for later energy needs in a form called glycogen. The amount your body can store as glycogen is somewhat limited. If you still have more glucose in your system, specialized cells start converting it to fat for storage.

Let's talk about water weight: Glycogen is heavy to store. It takes between 3 and 4 grams of water to store one gram of glycogen. If you are a carb-lover who keeps your glycogen tank full, you could be carrying up to 10 pounds of this water weight in your muscles and liver just to store all this glycogen. It's important to understand this in order to understand short-term variations in your weight. If you move into a fasting mode, you'll lose much of this water weight as you move into that ketonic (fat burning) state. If you move out of a fasting mode and refill your tanks, that weight can come back. If and as you weigh yourself frequently, you should learn not to attach too much significance to the ups and downs caused by water weight. Real weight loss is reduction of fat, and real weight gain is an increase in stored fat (or muscle).

Let's talk about the Adkins diet: Lots of folks who have gone on the Adkins low-carb diet get very excited at the outset, because they lose a lot of weight quickly. Unfortunately, this often comports with water weight connected to your body having a reduced inventory of glycogen. The permanent change in your diet (eliminating carbs) permanently reduces stored glycogen. After that water weight "goes away", then comes the hard part: losing fat. This is why so many persons you talk to get excited about the Adkins diet at first, but then after a few weeks lose interest and enthusiasm.

Let's talk about the often-cited "Glycemic Index": Even if you are not an Adkins follower, you've probably heard that it's good to eat carbs with some kind of glycemic index, but you never can quite remember if it's good to go for "high" or "low" (I'll answer that). Glycemic index is a great tool to help you think about carbs.

Glycemic index is measured by giving test subjects the exact same grams of carbohydrates delivered in different foods (for example peas, or potatoes) and seeing what impact eating those foods have on blood sugar over the next two hours. The impact of these foods on your blood sugar is compared to the impact of just eating pure glucose in the same clinical subjects (the same people). Foods with a low glycemic index, deliver blood sugar slowly (and will continue to deliver after the 2-hour test), foods with a high glycemic index deliver it more quickly, and look more like "pure glucose" in the test. So bottom line is that low glycemic index is the GOOD one. If you eat something with a high glycemic index, you'll get too much sugar too fast, your body will overproduce insulin, some of that glucose will be stored as fat, and you will crash and feel hungry again. Foods with lower glycemic index deliver glucose more slowly for a couple of reasons, mainly related to the need to perform extra metabolism to get to glucose, and also the fact that good slow carbs will have that starch matrixed inside insoluble fiber which takes your body more time to solve. Pure glucose has a glycemic index of 100. For actual foods, anything with a glycemic index over 70 is very high, and anything under 50 is low. Under 25 is great. To give you some real world examples, cabbage and asparagus have glycemic index under 20. Nuts and seeds generally have low glycemic indices. White potatoes can be close to 90.

OK, NOW WE'VE LEARNED A TON ABOUT CARBOHYDRATES IN TWO PAGES, LETS TALK ABOUT WHAT IT ALL MEANS.

Part of my objective in writing this book on reaching your ideal weight is to make it easy, and not to give you "too much to think about" with detailed diet plans, rules, and regimen's. So far the thread has gone as follows: being fat will kill you early, calculate your ideal weight, get a sense of how many calories you can eat per day, get comfortable with hunger, and fast regularly to drive your body into fat burning mode. I've shared some great information to inform and persuade you.

I hope that by talking about carbohydrates, I've made you feel smarter without giving you too much science, which will make you feel like you need a Ph.D. to follow a diet. Here's all you need to know about carbs in order to reach your ideal weight. Carbs are very energy dense. You only eat a little bit and you get a huge dose of calories. It's easy to overeat them. To make matters worse, if you eat them all at once, you'll get rebound hunger. You can eat a lot more vegetables meeting your daily calorie target than you can carbs. Think about how much grass a horse eats.

Carbs are not evil. You need available access to energy to function, and carbs are a possible source. So the idea is to simply eat fewer carbs than your instincts dictate, and eat carbs that deliver slowly (asparagus), over those that deliver fast (mashed potatoes). The FDA food plate is correct, it shows you keeping carbs at a quarter or less of your plate, and picking whole grains (lower glycemic index). Most of us, honestly, are "sedentary" or "low-active" on the scale in Chapter 3, yet most of us eat something like 300 grams of carbohydrates per day (1,200 calories). That's half the calories we need. 100 grams per day would be a better target. Keep in mind, a New York bagel can easily have 50 grams, and a soda can have 40 grams.

Carbohydrates are the only macronutrient that is not essential for life. You would die without protein or fat. Your body uses these to build its structures. Carbs are a quick source of energy. Nothing more. Your body can also make energy from fat and even protein. So it would be ok to eat zero carbs. Remember that. Think of carbs like a treat, and use them in moderation.

Carbohydrates: easy to overeat and the only macronutrient whose absence won't kill you. A little is ok. None is fine too.

So, as you'll learn in the last chapter, "Putting it All Together", I don't advocate obsessively counting calories or grams of anything unless you enjoy it and it helps YOU. Most of us don't have that kind of stamina. You'll drive yourself nuts and fall off your program. So here is what you need to do. When you see a carbo-bomb sitting on your plate, push some of it aside. Keep those carbs on the corner of your plate. And pick carbs that deliver slowly whenever possible. Pick brown rice over white rice. ENJOY carbs to give you energy. Eat some rice or potatoes every day if you like them. View them as a treat. A few bites of mashed potatoes. Binge once or twice a week with all the pizza you want, or dinner rolls at Cracker Barrel. Treat a soda like a desert or a rare treat you have every month or two. You'll enjoy it more anyway. Enjoy your carbs and make them meaningful.

On Gluten

Gluten. It would be disingenuous in the current era to write a short survey on nutrition and carbohydrates without addressing the issue of gluten. While gluten is not a carbohydrates (it's a protein), you get it from eating our classic carbohydrate: wheat. Gluten is the name for two glue-like proteins in whole wheat that give certain foods great glue-ey consistency and chewiness. As you read above, there are several reasons not to gorge yourself on carbohydrates, especially simple high-glycemic index carbs that give you more blood sugar than you can handle. Unfortunately, avoiding gluten isn't one of the good reasons to avoid carbohydrates. Read on.

Somewhere between 0.5% and 1.0% of the population has a genetic disorder called *celiac disease* (Celiac Disease Foundation, 2015). Celiac disease is an auto-immune disease. Its symptoms occur because the immune system identifies one of the metabolic products of gluten metabolism as an enemy and attacks the lining of the intestine. This causes atrophy of the lining of the small intestine, poor digestion, and all kinds of gastro-intestinal symptoms. Over long periods, it can cause intestinal cancer. There is only one treatment for celiac disease: life-long avoidance of grains containing gluten (wheat, rye, barley).

In addition to celiac disease, there is a condition that also can cause reaction to carbohydrates: *wheat allergy*. While prevalence of wheat allergy is under debate, it appears to be even more rare than celiac disease, affecting maybe 0.2% of the population. Further, it appears to be most commonly a pediatric allergy that resolves in later childhood. There are about 27 potential allergens in wheat, so even if you do have a positive test for wheat allergy, it doesn't mean you have an allergy to gluten.

Finally there is a characterization called "gluten sensitivity" that has been postulated in media and nutrition press, and is much discussed. There is no consensus yet that "gluten sensitivity" is a real condition separate and distinct from the known gluten sensitivity of celiac disease. If "gluten sensitivity" is real, and also distinct from celiac disease it has not been characterized with respect to cause or symptoms, and for example, in medical diagnostics there are not yet medical diagnostic codes assigned to this condition. In other words, the jury is out as to whether this condition, distinct from celiac disease, is real.

There is a furor going on in the manufactured food industry of removing gluten from wheat-based foods, or marketing foods that don't already contain gluten as "healthy" because they are "gluten-free". Here is the bottom line to cut through all of the hype. *If you think you might have celiac disease or a wheat allergy, see a doctor and get tested. If you don't have any symptoms, it may be worthwhile to limit carbohydrates, but you have absolutely no reason to worry about gluten, avoid gluten, or pay extra for foods that are positioned as gluten free.*

FAT

This has been one of the hardest sections of this manual for me to write concisely. The problem is that "fat" describes a whole bunch of non-water soluble compounds in our diets, and their use and metabolism in our body is horrendously complicated. Further, much has changed in what we know and what we thought we knew about fat in the last 25 years. We used to think that since fats are easily stored as body fat, eating them makes you fat. In the last decade however, this false idea has been thoroughly dismissed. While some fats may be unhealthy, overall the right fats can be considered health food, and an essential part of the human diet.

Fortunately, eating healthy fats is not difficult. The goal in writing this brief overview is to educate you. Quantity of food (calories) determines your weight, not the mix of fats you eat. If you are obese, reaching your ideal weight is more important for your health than getting engrossed by the science of fat. If you care about long term heart health, you should understand more about fat.

In nutrition, not only are fats sources of energy, but they are also sources of structure for cells and membranes, are required for neurological function, and of course act as a storage depot for extra energy. Too much fat or the wrong kind of fat may lead to heart disease and cardiovascular disease. Fats are fraught with benefits and peril, but actually much more on the benefits side. It's not hard to learn what to avoid.

First, fats don't make you fat. Eating too much makes you fat. The trend about 20 years ago for "low-fat" foods is seen now by some epidemiologists as a public health disaster. It caused people to eat more carbohydrates which increased obesity in the US. Fats don't make you fat, but unhealthy fats can harm your vascular health (heart and circulatory system). So the only goal you should have around fat is to try to eat a good quantity of the healthier fats. In fact, for a healthy person, close to half your calories can come from fat.

To try to lay this all out, I am going to start with a brief chat on cholesterol (balls made by your body to transport fat around your body), and then talk about the fats you actually eat from saturated to trans- to unsaturated (and suggest which ones to eat lots of. Finally I will mention triglycerides, which are a form of fat that circulates in your blood that can be turned into energy. At that point you'll have everything you need to understand fat's impact on your health.

Cholesterol. I start out talking about **cholesterol**, because most of the health threats caused by eating fat come from your body's propensity for making too much cholesterol, which can be a heart buster. Your liver needs fat to make cholesterol. For the purist, cholesterol is not actually a fat. It's grouped with fats in a category called "lipids". Lipids are compounds that won't dissolve in water (think of fat floating to the top in homemade soup).

Cholesterol is essential for your health and biological function. It's a waxy substance that occurs in every cell. It is needed to produce Vitamin D, and it is used in structural components throughout your body, in membranes, linings, and structures that need impermeability and flexibility. It is needed to produce certain digestive enzymes. It's also believed to be critical in the production of memory and in neurological function. It's essential for life every second and it's hardly just a "bad fat". Unfortunately because almost nobody has too little of it, it gets a horrible reputation as a heart clogger.

Your liver makes cholesterol every single day – in fact, unless you eat an extraordinary amount of "dietary cholesterol" (think egg yolks), your liver probably makes more cholesterol by itself than the amount you get from food. This is precisely why there is still not great consensus on what causes high cholesterol: you make the stuff yourself. What causes you to make too much? Your genes or what you ate?

And here comes an important analogy similar to the impact of a surge in your blood sugar on insulin: When you eat a lot of certain fats, it's believed that may cause your liver to make too much cholesterol. Your liver doesn't seem to have a great handle on how much cholesterol your cells need. It just sends the cholesterol out to your cells and lets them decide what they need. This creates a huge problem when we gorge ourselves: if there is a surfeit of cholesterol circulating in the blood, it starts to deposit as structural material on blood vessel walls. It constricts those vessels, and over time becomes hard and nasty. Eventually, pockets of it can rupture like a pimple popping, causing clotting and a complete blockage of coronary arteries: a heart attack.

How is cholesterol sent into the bloodstream? Remember I said that cholesterol is not water soluble – so the liver packages it into a protein ball so it can float around in the blood. There are two kinds of protein balls: the infamous **low density lipoprotein (LDL)** ball ("bad" cholesterol) and the famous **high density lipoprotein (HDL)** ball ("good" cholesterol). These are the two key components of your blood cholesterol. (Another bad cholesterol called VLDL is also in your lab counts.)

Here is the important fact about the relationship between LDL proteins and HDL proteins: Since your liver mostly sends cholesterols out to the extremities without a good handle on requirements, you have those HDL cholesterol containers to come by and pick up the extra. HDLs act like a scavenger, collecting un-needed cholesterol, and bringing it back to the liver for disposal. HDL's are the cholesterol clean-up crew, which prevent cholesterol over-accumulation in your arteries. This is why your doctor no longer cares about your total cholesterol when he reads your **cholesterol count**. If you have 250 (mg/dl) blood cholesterol (a high total) but most of that is HDL, you might be the healthiest guy in the world. So your **total cholesterol count** is comprised of your bad LDLs and your good HDLs.

When you see your doctor, if your cholesterol counts are good, you really don't need to worry too much about how much cholesterol you eat and the kinds of fats you eat. If you are at your ideal weight and you are maintaining your ideal weight I would be very surprised if your doctor tells you that you have high cholesterol.

If you still do have high cholesterol, it makes sense to think about the types of fat you eat. Most experts agree reducing saturated fats in your diet helps solve the problem. Saturated fats come from eating dairy (egg, milk, cheese) or fatty cuts of meat like beef, chicken, and pork (see the **Table 11**). You always hear that red meat is the villain, but fatty cuts of pork and chicken also have lots of saturated fat. If your cholesterol is high, you want to substitute healthy fats (olive oil, oily fish, nuts) for unhealthy fats (fatty meat and dairy). Not hard to remember. I'll talk slightly more about this in the next section explaining unsaturated fats (healthy), trans fats, and saturated fats (unhealthy).

The most important thing for you to do about cholesterol is see your doctor once a year and get him to test your cholesterol. If your bad cholesterol (LDL) is over 190 (mg/dl), you are considered at very high risk for heart disease. You should look for a score around 100. If your good cholesterol (HDL) is under 40, your risk is also elevated. Try for the good stuff to be 50 or better. Remember though, if you have a huge score on the good cholesterol, higher levels of the bad cholesterol are ok. So ask your doc if you aren't sure.

The next obvious question would be, ***should I take drugs if my cholesterol is high***? There are a couple of drugs called "statins" that lower your blood's bad cholesterol level by inhibiting an enzyme your body needs to make it. Some critics have argued that while there's proof that statins lower your blood cholesterol, there's not proof yet that they reduces death from heart disease. The reality is that they almost certainly do prevent heart disease. So the only issue is that if you take them, you need to take them permanently, and they do have side effects like muscle pain and weakness, so you have to decide if you want to live with that.

Two new anti-bad-cholesterol drugs came on the market in 2015. These drugs block a protein which would normally prevent the liver from eliminating bad cholesterol. The expectation is that these drugs are more tolerable (less side effects) than statins. The downside is that these new drugs need to be injected, may cost $1,000 per month, and may have long-term side effects that aren't yet known. So the bottom line is that drugs probably work if you can tolerate the side effects; however, if you reach your ideal weight, it's unlikely that you need them. For the cost of a cheap book, why not try that first?

Dietary fats – Saturated to Unsaturated. To be precise, dietary fats in isolation are called "**fatty acids**". Most dietary fat consists of three fatty acids are be chained together with something called a glycerol molecule, forming a bundle. These packaged fats are called "**triglycerides**". While an abundance of dietary fats come in the form of triglycerides, we can't really take those triglycerides across the wall of our intestines. So we break them apart into fatty acids, and rebuild triglycerides on the other side. This section is about what we eat. The next section talks about the triglycerides your body re-makes which circulate in your blood. We eat dietary fats in everything from nuts and oils, to fish, to dairy products, and other kinds of meat.

So how do I know what fats are healthy? Use **Table 11** below. You'll see the last three columns are fats ordered by degree of "hydrogenization". Fats have carbon and hydrogen. Fats that hold all the hydrogen they can are called "**saturated**" (column 2). Fats that don't hold all the hydrogen they can are called "unsaturated fats" (column 4). The **unsaturated fats** are the healthy ones, and the best examples of good sources are olive and canola oil, oily fish, and the fat in nuts.

The "**saturated fats**" are the ones that hold all the hydrogen they can and are solid at room temperature. Many experts, including the American Heart Association, call saturated fats "unhealthy" because they seem to encourage your body to make more of that LDL (bad) cholesterol.

Table 11 shows you what foods to avoid if you want to reduce saturated fats. Between the second column and the last column of the table is a column labelled **"trans-fats"**. They are kind of half way between saturated fats (solid) and unsaturated fats (liquid). Trans-fats are fats that are almost always man-made in a factory (trace amounts do occur in meat and dairy). They are made by adding back some of the missing hydrogen from those healthy liquid unsaturated fats. The reason food scientists developed this "innovation" was that you get a consistency for your fat between liquid and solid – a nice creamy material perfect for fake butter, canned frosting, and factory-made baked goods. Such fats also last longer on store shelves.

Fat	Cholesterol	Saturated Fats	Trans Fats	Unsaturated Fats
Hyrdogenization	NA	Full	Partial	Partial
Description at Room Temp	NA	Solid	Creamy	Liquid
Healthiness	Neutral	Neutral	Deadly	Generally Healthy
When to Eat	Routinely in Correct Moderation	Routinely in Correct Moderation	Never	Whenever you want
Examples	Eggs (highest) Animal Fats Butter Fried Chicken Steak Shellfish	Milk Cheese Butter Animal Fats Steak Pork Chicken Palm, Coconut Oil	Manufactured Baked Goods Pre-Made Frostings Margarine Hard to Find in Any Foods Today	Oily Fish Salmon, Trout, Tuna Nuts Almonds, Walnuts, Pecans, Peanuts Healthy Oils Olive, Canola

Table 11 – Lipids you'll encounter in your diet, and how to evaluate them.

What we did not conclude until the 1990's was that trans-fats seem to be horrendous contributors to heart disease, perhaps causing 30,000 deaths per year (W Willet, 1994). That's as many as die in car crashes in the US. The reason these fats are so dangerous is that – again for reasons not completely understood – trans-fats seem to cause your blood levels of LDL bad cholesterol to go up and HDL good cholesterol to go down. A double whammy for heart health. While there seems to be controversy around the impact of saturated fats on LDL cholesterol, there seems to be little controversy about trans-fats, for which show strong statistical associations to heart disease, even though underlying mechanisms are not understood.

It's debatable whether I should have mentioned trans-fats in this chapter, because food makers have almost completely removed them from manufactured food, and quick serve restaurants have taken them out of frying oil. Food labels can call trans-fat "zero" if trans-fat represents less than 0.5 grams per serving – so if you are worried, check the ingredients for "partially hydrogenated" oils. Trans-fats should not be considered safe to eat at any level and you should strive to consume zero.

Finally, let's talk about those healthy "**unsaturated fats**". These are the fats in the last column of Table 11. The good news here is you can eat these fats with impunity. They seem to invoke little controversy. Most doctors today will tell you that if you have high cholesterol, don't eat less fat. Replace cholesterol (eggs, butter, shellfish), and saturated fats (meat and cheese) with healthy fats. (DON'T replace those less unhealthy fats with carbs!) Again, you can find the healthy fats in olive oil, oily fish (salmon, tuna), nuts, avocados, and plant oils such as canola oil and sunflower oil.

The only thing you are likely to find yourself "controversial" in the area of healthy fats is that there are a couple of different kinds and some are seen as "better" than others. In healthy unsaturated fats you find Omega-3 and Omega-6 fatty acids. Certain of the Omega-3 and Omega-6 fatty acids are called "essential fats" because your body needs them and can't make them. Omega-3 is believed to be the healthiest of all, having strong anti-oxidant (repair) and anti-inflammatory properties, in addition to being heart healthy and lowering bad cholesterol. Omega-6 is believed to have heart-healthy properties as well, but not as powerfully as Omega-3's. Since both types of fatty acid are metabolized by the same enzyme, some specialists say too much Omega-6 "crowds out" the more potent Omega-3. There are also some complaints that grain fed beef has more Omega-6 to the detriment of Omega-3. If you are a fanatic about Omega-3, use olive oil and eat natural salmon, otherwise this controversy is way too specious for you to consider. Especially if you are overweight.

The State of Science on Saturated Fats

The idea that the prevalent fat in meats and dairy – saturated fat – is unhealthy is ingrained in all of us. So you may be incredulous to learn that there is not universal agreement on the belief that a diet high in saturated fats has a long-term effect of raising LDL cholesterol. Over the past 40 years a few studies have seemed to show that persons eating diets high in saturated fat have (again meats and dairy) have more heart disease. Often, the "American Diet" is compared with the "Mediterranean Diet" – more olive oil, less cheese and red meat – and lower incidence of heart disease in those populations.

There are a couple of problems with this. First there is no scientific understanding of what triggers your liver to make more cholesterol from the fat you eat, no confirmed theory on why saturated fat would cause your body to make more cholesterol, and no understanding of what mechanism causes a high ratio of the bad LDL, versus the good HDL which cleans up cholesterol returning it to the liver for metabolism. If genetics play a strong role, that could contribute to racial differences as much as diet does. Maybe those Mediterraneans have a genetic propensity to have low bad cholesterol! In fact, all the raw materials your liver would need to make cholesterol are available in the other "healthy fats" – so we really don't know what might cause the liver to make more cholesterol, or more bad cholesterol just because you ate saturated fat.

There is even persuasive evidence that eating too much sugar can cause high triglycerides and high cholesterol even if you don't eat a lot of fat / saturated fat. A surprising study published in the journal Obesity cut the level of sugar in obese children from around 30% of calories to 10% of calories, and saw return of triglycerides and cholesterol from highly elevated levels to normal levels. The most surprising factor was that the study lasted just nine days (Robert H. Lustig, 2015).

Without settled science, we are left relying on large observational studies that attempt to track what people eat, and then observe how they fared. These studies have a hard time accounting for how genetic differences might impact outcomes. To throw further confusion into the mix, a huge meta-analysis of other studies which was completed in 2014 and included half a million subjects was inconclusive as to whether the diet high in saturated fat contributed to heart disease (Siri-Tarino PW, 2010). Critics say that the studies that do show a positive association between saturated fat consumption and LDL are too small and too short-term to be conclusive.

To add a little more dimension to the debate, it should be noted that saturated fat includes any of the family of fats that are completely saturated with hydrogen. There are at least 5 separate kinds, and there are suspicions that Stearic and Lauric saturated fats (found in chocolate, coconut oil, and meats) may be relatively benign (or "good"), while Myristic and Palmitic saturated fats (found in meat, dairy, and palm oil) may be "bad" actors (Katz., 2015).

The science isn't settled and I do not mean to wade into this debate, especially as it becomes more complex, and we keep subdividing our fats into smaller and smaller classifications. So what should a fat-concerned eater do?

1. Have your blood lipids (cholesterol, triglycerides) tested.
2. Reach your ideal weight
3. Have your lipids tested again. Are they ok?
4. If not, try avoiding meats high in fat and dairy products.
5. Have your lipids tested. Are they ok?
6. Consider medication.

Really I hope that most of you are in good shape after step 2!

Triglycerides. The last topic we need to loop back on to finish the discussion of fat is **triglycerides**. Remember I said this form of fat is comprised of three fatty acids shackled together with a glycerol molecule. This package is an efficient way for your body to move fuel fat around (as opposed to structure fat – cholesterol – moved around in those LDL/HDL balls). Your liver throws some triglycerides inside those LDL/HDL balls with the cholesterol. You also have triglycerides circulating directly in your blood. Just as glucose (which comes from your carbs) is a great source of energy, the fatty acids in triglycerides are also fairly easily used by cells for energy. As triglycerides circulate in your blood, your cells grab them and either use them for energy, or convert them for permanent storage as body fat, depending on whether or not you ate too much. Fat is an important source of energy, and healthy persons may get 30- to 50% of their daily energy from fat. Triglycerides are the fuel packs that move this energy around.

I told you not to hyper-focus on the fats you eat if your cholesterol LDL and HDL numbers are healthy. When you get lipid blood tests done, another number they will give you is your triglycerides. If your triglycerides are below150 (mg/dl) that's generally considered ok. If they are higher, this is considered by some experts to be *an even more potent marker of arteriosclerosis and heart disease risk than high cholesterol*. A specific mechanism for triglycerides causing heart disease isn't identified; however, a very strong statistical correlation has been seen between high triglycerides and heart disease. High triglycerides are more of a marker for heart disease than a cause. Wow. Lipidologists can puzzle on this, but I can give you a little insight: if you eat too much, your liver is going to package as much of that excess fat as it can into triglycerides and send it into your bloodstream. Your cells can't keep up with soaking it all up, packaging, and turning it into body fat. Your cells gets backed up on the rate it can turn these bundles it into body fat. Your tissues are like a wet sponge for triglycerides: constantly trying to soak up more and put them all away. The amount stranded in your blood are high. So here's some good advice if your triglycerides are very high: You are eating too much! That's why I think there is such a strong correlation. People with the high triglycerides are usually the fat people.

FATS - SUMMARY

That was a lot of information. So let me restate the key points. Don't avoid fat – it's as good a source of energy as carbohydrates. Have your cholesterol checked. If your bad cholesterol is too high, get to your ideal weight and see if that solves the problem. Your cholesterol problem may be an "eating too much" problem, rather than a dietary fats mix issue. If you've reached your ideal weight and your cholesterol is still high, try eating less saturated fat, especially fatty meat and dairy, and see if it helps. If your cholesterol is good, don't spend too much time thinking about fat. Have no regrets about eating healthy unsaturated fats.

PROTEIN

While nothing is simple when it comes to human metabolism, thankfully, explaining the role of proteins on nutrition is much easier than explaining fats. When you eat proteins, your body basically breaks them down into a soup of amino acids. Amino acids are the building blocks of proteins, and your body uses these components to reassemble the protein material eaten into the proteins it needs to perform its business.

There are about 20 different amino acids. Eleven of them are "non-essential" meaning your body can make them if it's short. Nine of the amino acids are "essential" meaning your body can't make them and needs to find them in your diet. Eating protein as meat provides all the essential amino acids. If you are a vegetarian, you have to work harder to get all the essential amino acids your body needs: you can't get "complete" protein from a single food unless that food is meat.

If it's possible to rank-order two items that are 100% necessary for human existence, proteins are more essential than fats (that's silly, you'd die without either one). Proteins are the structural building blocks of many tissues including muscle and other organs. Proteins have functional biological roles in cellular communication and interaction. Proteins on the surfaces of cells communicate with other cells, send biological signals, and act as sentries to determine what may enter cells. Proteins are also the stuff of enzymes, which drive and catalyze chemical reactions that are the fabric of life.

Proteins are not an important source of energy in your body. If your body has access to carbohydrates, it will recruit those first for energy, then fat, and finally protein. Recall that carbohydrates have about 4 calories of energy per gram, and fat has 9 calories per gram. Protein also has 4 grams of energy per calorie, but it's harder for your body to get at that energy. If your body is digesting its own muscle tissue for energy, it's usually considered a sign of starvation (though your body may use the protein you eat for energy without starvation).

Your body will digest dietary protein for energy if you don't supply it enough carbohydrates or fat. All protein contains nitrogen. The process of digesting protein for energy is called "deamination", and involves your body stripping the nitrogen-bearing ammonium off of the amino acids. This has the impact of converting the protein to a sugar-like substance that is ultimately harvested for energy like a carbohydrate.

Lean protein is something you can eat relatively guilt-free. Most guidelines tell you to eat one-third of your body weight in grams. For example, if you weigh 150 pounds, you would eat about 50 grams a day. This will provide you with about 10% of your caloric needs for the day (50 grams * 4 calories / gram = 200 calories). If you have reached the stage of your weight loss program where you are adding muscle, you should eat much more protein. It's ok to have as much of a third of your calories come from protein. A strength-training rules is to try to eat your weight in grams of calories – i.e. if you weigh 150 pounds, eat 150 grams.

I will talk about exercise more in the next chapter, but if you do engage in strength training, your body can use extra amino acids to build muscle for 24 to 48 hours after your strength-training work out. You need to make sure this protein is available. In terms of adding muscle, supplying the raw material is as important as working out.

Finally, if you have high cholesterol, remember meat can payload a lot of saturated fat, which is suspected to increase that "bad cholesterol". Most people think of chicken as kind of a "safe" lean meat, but a chicken thigh, even with the skin off, can have up to twice as much fat as a lean sirloin – so be careful in focusing on lean meats (chicken breasts, pork, fish). Check a calorie counting site, such as *My Fitness Pal* if you aren't sure.

ALCOHOL

Alcohol can be characterized as the "fourth" macronutrient following carbohydrates, fat, and protein. For many of us, it is a "food group": a good deal of folks get a substantial fraction of their calories from it. Many of us like to have a cocktail or two to relax and feel social. Alcohol is a food, and it is a source of energy. As a macronutrient, its closest analogy is probably the carbohydrate, because it is a decent source of energy, and doesn't have other important nutritive or biochemical functions.

Alcohol has about 7 calories of energy per gram. Your body needs to know how to metabolize alcohol even if you don't drink: certain normal metabolic processes have small amounts of alcohol as a byproduct. When you drink alcohol, your body breaks it down at a steady rate. Your body has to "throttle" the metabolism of alcohol, because one of the metabolic products of its breakdown – acetylaldehyde – is toxic and it can't be allowed to reach dangerous levels. Digest alcohol too quickly and you will poison yourself. Acetylaldehyde is broken down to a vinegar-like compound which is digested like a sugar.

Scores of observational studies have suggested that moderate drinking leads to better health and longevity. Many of these studies relate to the drinking of wine. The mechanism for this health effect is not fully identified, but it is believed that alcohol may have worthwhile antioxidant / anti-inflammatory effects that help your metabolism repair and recover. Most of the observational studies on alcohol suggest the greatest benefit is around one drink per day on average or a little less. Excessive drinking can have horrible health impacts. One of the worst is fatty liver and cirrhosis, but excess alcohol, can also damage the brain, the pancreas, weaken the heart muscle, cause high-blood pressure, and stroke. Ouch.

So if you drink, moderation is very important – a little may be healthy, a lot is deadly. Also, for your ideal weight, a lot is deadly. A lot of people focus on calories and diet in an attempt to lose weight, but "give themselves a pass" on a few drinks over the weekend, which may amount to six or seven drinks. A glass of wine, a shot of whiskey, and a beer each have about 150 calories in a serving. With the hard liquor, if that is mixed with fruit juice in a fancy cocktail, you can easily double the calories per drink. So I'm not telling you not to drink. I'm just telling you to include it in your allowed rewards (see Chapter 8) without disregarding its calorie count.

So if you go into each weekend sober and come out on the other side having had 7 drinks, you could be adding 1,400 calories to your regimen. That's nearly an eighth day of eating. It counts! Damn, no wonder you can't lose weight. So if you use alcohol, use it in moderation and consider it in your calories. One drink a day means you need to reduce your food calories by a couple of hundred.

ON THE CORRECT COMPOSITION OF YOUR DIET (CARBS/FAT/PROTEIN)...

There is a great deal written in the field of nutrition about dietary mix, and oceans of suggestions that your mix can help you lose weight. While a healthy diet contains a balanced mix of carbohydrates, fat, and protein, the reality is that only the amount of calories you consume and your activity substantially determine weight gain.   The mix only matters if you find eating certain things helps you eat less overall.

In looking at popular diet discussions and trends, you'll find arguments that since carbohydrates and fat are ready sources of energy, while proteins are not as accessible (remember proteins require "deamination" before they can be used for energy), your body has to work harder to digest protein. As this argument goes, for each calorie of protein consumed, you'll have fewer excess calories to turn into energy or fat. This argument is very appealing to those of us who like to eat a lot but need to lose weight. The hope is that you can eat more calories worth of protein with less weight gain.

Unfortunately, there is not good evidence that this free-ride is meaningful. In an excellent article on the impact of energy imbalance on body weight, which is published in the prestigious journal *Lancet*, Kevin Hall (Kevin D Hall, 2011) and six other scientists describe the results of a detailed model they have developed to simulate the movement of calorie energy through our metabolic processes, and how it drives the creation and destruction of tissue (fat, protein, etc). Because our metabolism is complex, and the mix of what we eat impacts how energy is stored (fat, glycogen, etc.) there is a theoretical argument that for the same calories, diet composition can impact weight. The reality, however that there is a lot of "cancellation of error" among outcomes that relating to the mix of what you eat. Citing at least 40 different scientific studies and journal articles, Hall concludes that there is no evidence that your dietary mix has any material impact on weight gain or loss. In other words for all reasonable purposes a calorie really is a calorie is a calorie, just as I first asserted in Chapter 3.

So let's talk about what is a reasonable dietary mix of carbohydrate, fat and protein. As you know, this book is not for banning carbohydrates. They are a great source of accessible energy, especially when you choose carbohydrates with a low glycemic index (so they deliver energy slowly). But please remember, that carbohydrates (and alcohol) are the only macronutrient that you don't actually need to survive, and they are a very dense form of calories (and also very delicious) so it is very easy for you to eat too much. When you think about eating carbs, if you are overweight, your risk of diabetes may not be driven per se by the fraction of carbs you eat, but rather that since you are eating too much you are eating too many carbs.

Table 12 shows you reasonable range of healthy mix among the macronutrients. If you are going to hit the low end of the range on any of these nutrients, it should be carbohydrates. Your body can use fat to make energy, eating too many carbohydrates increases risk of diabetes, and as we've discussed carbohydrates can have low satiety impact, i.e. you are hungry again sooner. (Chapter 4 discussed that you do have to learn to be comfortable with hunger, but why make it harder than necessary?)

Macronutrient	Energy Mix (% total calories)
Carbohydrates	30- to 45%
Fat	30- to 45%
Protein	10- to 35%

Table 12 – Reasonable Range for Dietary Mix.

On lean protein, the range is wide. Many public health sources recommend you eat about 1/3 of your body weight in grams of daily protein. IE – if you weigh 150 pounds, eat 50 grams of lean protein per day. As I mentioned earlier, this works out to be about 10% of your total calories. However, if you are engaging in strength training you need much more protein to add muscle, and many sources (including me) recommend that you eat your body weight in grams of protein – i.e. if you weigh 150 pounds, eat 150 grams per day, or about 30% of your calories. If you are significantly overweight, I don't recommend you engage in strength training until you are well on your weigh to losing your excess weight. Adding muscle while cutting fat can be confusing, and you need to learn to lose weight before you start mixing in muscle mass. As you start to lose weight, it's ok to be lower in the protein range.

ON POPULAR DIETS …

This book is written to tell you how to reach your ideal weight, not to tell you exactly what you have to eat, because the fact is that there are a whole variety of diets that will provide you health and nutrition. Many diet books have scores of pages telling you exactly what to eat to lose weight, including 100's of recipes, and daily meal plans. I believe these treatments focus you on the wrong discipline and are extremely difficult for you to implement. Few can stay with them for very long because there are too many variables around the facts, circumstances, and conditions of your lifestyle, how and where you eat.

Also if you do great all-day by following a canned diet plan, assiduously preparing the meals in a prescriptive recipe book, and weighing portions before consumption, and then you have a little 500 calorie mini-binge right before you go to bed, you have a day with zero progress. While 95% of your focus and effort for the day went in to the prescribed menu, 100% of the problem came from that last 30 minutes. So we'll talk about this more in Chapter 8, but it's much more effective for you to weigh yourself frequently than it is to weigh your food frequently.

That being said, there are many diet programs that have very nutritious and healthful guidelines, and a few that are famous enough that they are worth mentioning here. There are other very popular diets that I'm not addressing, but this brief discussion should give you a basis to evaluate other commercial plans.

There are many different diets that are healthy, and the usual pitfall is the mistake of thinking that eating these healthy diets will necessarily help you with your weight. Once again, we are back to the truism that how much you eat, not what you eat, determines your weight. If you need more specificity of *what* to eat, it is worth evaluating a couple of commercial programs. If they help you stay disciplined, go for it! Remember always, if you are overweight, first and most important is to learn to manage *how much* you eat.

A kind of granddaddy of weight focused diets is ***The South Beach Diet***. This diet was developed by a cardiologist, Dr. Arthur Agatson, in the 1990's and first published in 2003. The *South Beach Diet* is so powerful because it is so sensible. In the prescription, there is an early phase of the diet with nearly zero carbohydrates, but after that, the diet summarily teaches the patient not to restrict carbohydrates or fats, but to eat "good" carbohydrates, and "good" fats, combined with lean proteins. Fruits and especially vegetables are always a good bet. Dr. Agatson was one of the first to identify the concept of good carbs and good fats, while many earlier diets focused on the mix of carbs, fats, and protein, with no deference to underlying foods.

A couple of caveats on the *South Beach Diet*. First, the early no-carb phase is focused on patients losing over 10 pounds in two weeks. An overweight person could lose over 10 pounds in 2 days on a zero-carb diet due to all the water weight associated with storing glycogen in the liver, but I don't believe this phase of the diet is necessary. Early rapid weight-loss can be confusing for a dieter or create false optimism, and in any event, the focus should be on reducing fat, not water weight. Second, because Dr. Agatson is a cardiologist, there definitely is a focus on avoiding saturated fat. As I discussed above, the connection between saturated fats and high heart-clogging cholesterol is not well established, and the best and most important way to determine how much attention you must pay to healthy fats is to have your own blood lipids (LDL, HDL, triglycerides) measured.

Ok, so obviously that brings us to the always controversial ***Atkins Diet***. The Atkins Diet is essentially a zero to very low carb diet that encourages eaters to load up on protein. If you read the section on nutrition above, you have concluded that lean protein and healthy (unsaturated) fats can be eaten with relative impunity, and that carbs are relatively dispensable and worthwhile to avoid... for Dr. Atkins, so far so good. The diet also seems to impel eaters not to worry about the saturated fats that may be payloaded in a meaty high-protein diet. This has led some to conclude, that on an Atkins Diet you may lose weight in the short term, but you'll be dead by 55 of a heart attack.

The Atkins diet isn't an unhealthy diet if your cholesterol is ok (again the only way to see if you might have a problem with unhealthy fat is to have your blood lipids tested). However the diet does come with a lot of caveats. First, the diet starts out with zero carb phase that moves to low carb phases. The aim is to force your body into a ketonic state (so that you are burning fat), and it aims to maintain that state. For optimal health, ability to clean and repair, and minimizing inflammation, your body should cycle through all its metabolic states like a car shifting gears. Regularly fasting or periodically eliminating carbs will also cycle you through ketosis, and do it routinely, rather than at the beginning of a "diet". Next, the diet is fairly complex – it has you eliminating carbs and then adding back limited certain carbs along numerous "rungs". You have to pay attention to "net carbs" in what you eat, and some versions have you monitoring your urine for ketones. It is way too complex for most people to stay focused. Next, quick early weight lost by eliminating carbs is not loss of fat. Atkins eaters often get encouraged by early rapid weight loss and then lose enthusiasm. That's another reason why many drop this diet. Finally, clinical studies of weight loss with Atkins versus alternate diets of similar calories have not shown a meaningful advantage for Atkins in weight loss (not a surprise for you if you've read this far). Dr. Atkins own initial clinical study showed only a 0.1- to 2.9% more weight loss than on other standard diets (KA Gudzune, 2015). If this diet helps you stay focused and eat the correct amount of food *nothing wrong with that.* What works for you is what works. However, don't expect to be able to eat more calories without getting fat!

The last specific mention should go to the **paleo diet**, which was popularized in a 2002 book *the paleo diet* by Loren Cordain. The idea is that our digestion and metabolism evolved in the Paleolithic period from 2 million to 10,000 years ago, and that the agricultural revolution around 10,000 years ago introduced all kinds of foods that we are not well adapted to digest, especially wheat, other grains, starchy legumes (beans), and dairy. It is this mismatch between biology and food that contributes to obesity and a host of obesity related diseases.

The paleo diet is a healthy diet. It pushes lots of meat, lots of good fatty fish, and lots of high-fiber plant-based foods. Nothing wrong with that!

As always, there are a few caveats. It is evident that there were many different diets during the paleo period – some all plant based, some all meat based. There is no true "paleo" diet. Human metabolism is very well adapted to tackle a variety of foods. Eschewing beans and other starchy plant foods makes it a great deal of work to get your needed calories, especially if you are a vegetarian. If you don't eat dairy, you also need to be certain you get enough calcium. There isn't yet scientific evidence that this diet has specific biological benefits in weight loss or preventing disease. I also believe that it places unnecessary emphasis on the "Paleolithic authenticity" of protein sources and eschewing the omega-6 type of fat (farmed meat has more Omega 6). Some people who have GI diseases such as IBS (irritable bowel symptom) say that it helps them (no real science on this yet). Bottom line for the third time – if this diet helps you manage how much you eat or what you should eat, *nothing wrong with that.* The biggest impactor of your weight and health is how much you eat.

Finally, let's mention a couple of recent fasting-focused diet techniques: **"The 8-Hour Diet"** and **"The Every Other Day Diet"**. I think the foods recommended in these books are largely sensible, and that the recommendations to use fasting are critical (even if the format is different than what I recommend: a weekly 24-hour fast). The issue, as I discussed is that "The 8-Hour Diet" suggests its ok if you only are able to follow the program a few days a week, and its ok to eat as much as you want during your 8-hours. These waivers may enable you to make no progress whatsoever. The "Every Other Day Diet" suggests not only that you can eat as much as you want on feast days, but you can eat whatever you want. Considering that modern food can payload huge calorie density (a regular Big Gulp has as many calories as about 20 cups of cooked broccoli), the notion that you can eat whatever you want on alternate days is also a potential recipe for failure in my opinion. I think these concessions by the authors might be ways to market these books. People want to hear they can meet goals without sacrifice. If persons with gastric surgery can eat through a reduced stomach, a fat person with a free pass can certainly ruin a diet in 3 or 4 "cheat days" per week. As I will discuss more in Chapter 8 frequent rewards are important; however open-ended or unlimited rewards can't drive success.

A SIMPLE PRÉCIS ON NUTRITION – IN 9 STEPS

If you read this chapter, hopefully the last few sections gave you some education about the nutrition and this précis will serve as a review. If you skipped it, it's worth taking note of the few large and widely accepted principals that will ensure your diet is both healthy and also not an impediment to reaching your ideal weight. The following summary (précis) tells you all that you need to know if you have normal health.

1. ***Your Weight***: If you are concerned about your health, and you are **overweight** or **obese** your weight is the greatest imminent threat to your health, and any concerns about what you are putting into your body (organic non-GMO cereal versus plain old corn flakes) is a false drama. None of these food fads have been connected to health or to mortality. Your **weight** is determined by how much you eat, not what you eat. Find the correct amount of food to reach your ideal weight, and you have won 95% of the health and nutrition battle. (If you need more guidance than a sense of your correct calories to make sure you eat the right things, consider this: eating things that that are close to nature is a pretty fault-tolerant approach: fruits, vegetables, nuts, fatty fish. That's the easiest way for you to avoid making health mistakes. Fruits and vegetables in particular have low calorie density (you have to work hard to get fat eating them) and close-to-nature foods don't deliver pure sugar or starchy carbo bombs that send you soaring over a daily calorie objective. See Bullet 7 below).

2. ***Carbohydrates*** are a great source of energy, but they have pitfalls. They are a very dense source of calories, and to add insult to injury, if you eat dense starchy carbohydrates, your body over-produces insulin which causes a rebound hunger. So it's very easy to eat too much when you eat carbohydrates. To combat this eat carbs that deliver energy slowly ("low glycemic index") – which means whole grains, bran, oats, beans, etc. When you are exposed to the most delicious carbs – pizza, dinner rolls, white breads, potatoes, candy, and foods

with added sugar – just enjoy a little bit and push most to the side. Treat it like a dessert. Carbohydrates are the most dispensable nutrient: your body does not need them for structures or key chemical processes, and you can also get energy from fats. Eating none is fine.

3. **Fats:** Much is made of the issue of **fats**. Fats are a great source of energy, and your body needs them for structure and metabolic processes. We know that **unsaturated fats are healthy fats**, and you can eat a lot of them. These are canola and olive oil, fats in nuts, and fatty fish. Some people think **saturated fats** contribute to high blood cholesterol, so that these are unhealthy fats. Too much cholesterol in your blood clogs your arteries and can damage your heart. Saturated fats are found in fatty cuts of beef, chicken and other meats, plus dairy products (milk and cheese). The mechanism that would cause eating of saturated fats to drive up your blood cholesterol is not well understood, so you should have your **blood cholesterol checked**. Look at your LDL, HDL, and Triglycerides. Make sure they are in the healthy range shown on your lab report. If your numbers are healthy, you don't need be obsessed with what fats you eat. If your numbers are not healthy, get to your ideal weight, and have them checked again. They'll probably be fixed. If they are still out of range, eat more of the healthy fats, and reduce the fatty meat and dairy. Have them checked again. Still unhealthy? Consider medication. Never eat trans fats or partially hydrogenated oils (a man-made fat rarely but occasionally still found in mass market foods).

4. **Protein:** Your body needs **protein** to build new structures, repair and replace structures, and to drive cellular function and chemistry. Your body does not usually use protein as an energy source. Lean protein is a healthy food. Under ordinary conditions, you should eat at least 1/3 of your body weight in protein grams – your body needs that for repair and replacement. (For example, if you weigh 150 pounds, eat at least 50 grams per day.) If you are strength training or adding muscle, eat fully your body weight in protein grams. (For example, if you weigh 150 pounds, eat 150 grams per day.) You can eat protein pretty much guilt free, but remember it may be paired with unhealthy fats, which is a concern if you have high cholesterol. If you eat it in nuts or in fatty fish, you are eating it paired with healthy fat. If you eat it as chicken, remember that some fatty cuts of chicken (wings and thighs) can have as much or more saturated fat as fatty beef. Lean cuts of chicken, pork, and beef, in addition to fish, are good sources of protein.

5. **Alcohol:** You don't need alcohol, but some studies have shown that in moderation (1 drink per day or less) it can contribute to longevity and health. In excess it is horrible for your health – brain, liver, heart, connective tissue. So don't rationalize alcohol as a health drink. If you do drink, remember to include

it in your calorie estimates. It has a lot of calories. A serving (beer, wine, hard liquor) has 150 calories, and a cocktail can be double that. A few drinks with the guys after work more than erases any day's progress in dieting, so do that as an occasional reward, not three times per week.

6. ***Dietary Mix***: For your **dietary mix** there is no villain among carbohydrates, fat, and protein. Eaten the right way, all can contribute to health and energy. A good balance of macronutrients is having around 1/3 of your calories coming from fats, 1/3 of your calories coming from carbohydrates, and 1/3 coming from protein. Most people eat less protein, but don't let less than 15% of your calories come from protein, and again, eat your weight in protein grams if you are adding muscle. It's always ok to reduce carbs. If you do this, replace it with healthy unsaturated fats and lean protein.

7. ***Fruits and Vegetables:*** Eat lots – they are self-limiting if you want to reach an ideal weight. They have fairly low calories per unit weight, and they'll displace carbs and other things you eat which are denser in calories. (Remember the example of the Big Gulp soda having the same calories as 20 cups of cooked broccoli.) Vegetables contain a lot of micronutrients. In large volume, they are filling, so they are also a hunger busting technique. Fiber is good for your digestive track and believed to reduce risk of colon cancer. Fruits have sugar that can provide you energy. The sugar in fruits – fructose – isn't healthier than cane (regular) sugar, despite what you may hear. Nevertheless, it's worth driving a lot of the simple sugar in your diet away from added sugar (cake, candy, soda), and getting it from fruit – because it comes along with fiber, better absorption, more bulk per unit delivery, and a modality that helps you avoid craving too much sugar.

8. **Micronutrients – vitamins, minerals:** Vitamins, minerals and water are called micronutrients, because your body needs them for chemistry, but they don't have any calories. If you are eating lots of fruits and vegetables, you won't need to take any vitamin supplements. When you get your doctor do routine bloodwork to test your cholesterol, he'll also tell you if he sees any vitamin deficiencies.

9. **Micronutrients – water:** Hydration is important so your body can conduct its chemistry and get rid of waste. Stay hydrated. The aphorism that you should drink "eight 8 ounce glasses of water per day" is an old-wives tale and is not based on research or study. Your daily needs could be much more or less than this depending on your size and activity. If you are urinating every 2 to 3 hours, and your urine runs fairly clear, you are hydrated. If not, drink more. Respiration while asleep is the greatest ordinary dehydrator. You will always be dehydrated after a good night's sleep, so pound a couple of glasses of water

every morning. Only drink water. If you like orange juice, fruit punch, or sodas, have 1 or 2 of these types of beverages per week. Treat them in the same category as alcohol or a dessert – something you do occasionally as a reward.

Because there is evidence that certain patterns of eating may reduce the time you spend hungry, a lot of counterproductive focus in the weight-loss industry is based on what you eat. Your weight is the biggest impactor of your health – and your weight is not determined by what you eat. Only by how much you eat. There are many healthy diets out there if you need guidance on what to eat, but look to them if you need inspiration, not as weight loss advice. Good nutrition is fairly simple – eat a mix of healthy fat, protein, and carbohydrates. Eat lots of fruits and vegetables. There are lots of delicious foods that are healthy. Enjoy food in the right quantity and remember to give yourself frequent rewards.

Exercises – Chapter 6 *Nutrition*

If you internalized this chapter, you are an expert on best current thinking about nutrition.

1. Write down something you learned about each of the three main macronutrients in Chapter 5.

Carbohydrates	
Fats	
Proteins	

2. List three things your read in Chapter 5 about nutrition that you didn't know, or that surprised you.

1.	
2.	
3.	

3. List two things your read in Chapter 5 about nutrition that you didn't believe. Use google to investigate. Did your thinking change?

Initially Surprised Me	After Researching

4. Having read Chapter 5, list a few things you are thinking about changing in your diet that would be fairly easy to change.

1.	
2.	
3.	

Chapter 7 – Exercise

Here's the good news if you don't like to exercise: you don't have to exercise very much or very long to live at your ideal weight or enjoy most of the benefits of exercise. You don't have to adopt a new lifestyle. You don't have to get up at 4 AM before your family gets up so you can do an hour of high-intensity swimming. I know you've read about people who do this kind of stuff, or have neighbors or folks at work who train for triathlons. You get those little reminders of the workouts they do, and you vacillate between feeling a little guilty about how sedentary you are, and wanting to actually punch them in the face. Here's a little more good news: even if you will never be that triathlete, after you've been at it a few months with exercise, you usually will find you look forward to a quick exercise like any other guilty pleasure. It helps you extinguish anxiety and stress. It can be a little addictive for many people.

Here's the bad news if you really don't like to exercise: You have to exercise. You don't need to exercise a lot, but you need to exercise. You should do structured exercise 4 or 5 times per week. As I go through this brief discussion on exercise, I'm going to tell you why you must exercise, how you should exercise, and how much you should exercise. But let me get this out up front: I feel that exercise is mandatory. While it's theoretically possible for you to reach your ideal weight without exercise, it's so challenging and counterproductive, that I would characterize it as constructively impossible.

What I won't do in this book is give you complex exercise routines, charts, tables of set and reps, and schematics of various exercises. Here's why: in exercise for weight management it really doesn't matter very much what you do. The only two parameters that really matter are **time** and **intensity**. You have to invest a little bit of time, and you should try to reach a state of high intensity for at least few minutes each session, which I'll teach you how to do shortly. After that, you get to decide what you do, and what is most engaging or enjoyable for you. I'll give you some suggestions and point you where to find easy resources.

Let me caveat my general latitude in how you exercise by saying that strength training is a little more technical than general exercise. If you have poor muscularity, you should add muscle as you move closer to your ideal weight, and I will discuss briefly the right resources to help you work that into your exercise routine over time. If you are very heavy, strength training doesn't need to be a focus of the early stages of your path to success. We'll give you a tighter prescription of what to do shortly.

Here's what you are going to learn in this chapter:

- Why should I exercise? How does it help me reach ideal weight?
- How should I exercise if I am obese or very overweight?
- How should I exercise as I near my ideal weight?

When you are done reading this chapter, you'll know what you need to do, and you'll have the tools and ideas to incorporate exercise into your life without making wholesale changes, adopting a new lifestyle (unless you want to), living only for exercise, or facing the intimidation of showing up at a gym obese and untrained.

WHY SHOULD I EXERCISE?

That's actually a really good question. I've pounded home the idea that the most important factor for your overall health if you are overweight is reaching your correct weight. I've pounded home the idea that really two things matter for reaching that correct weight: the amount of calories you burn (your activity) and the amount of calories you consume. So how does exercise fit in?

The obvious answer would be that if you increase exercise, you increase calories burned in "activity" --- but hang on. I'm not going to recommend that you ever spend more than an hour a day in structured exercise (for the heaviest folks), and not even seven days a week, at that. If you are close to your ideal weight, 25 minutes can be enough.

For a very heavy person, most of that exercise will be simply walking, until you start to show progress, with a few minutes of high intensity motion during the hour. So how much does this exercise impact your activity (calories burned)?

Not much. An hour of walking for a mid-weight person is worth about 225 calories. And you just used up an entire hour of your time. You are unlikely to burn even this much. Laying aside a Chobani yogurt and a half cup of juice has the same impact on your caloric balance. You may say "Hey, that's walking, but walking is barely exercise". If, on the other hand, you run nine-minute miles for an entire hour (6.7 miles), you'll burn about 750 calories. Most people can't run 7 miles in an hour. For those that can, it's very hard work. Yet for your hour, you only burned the calories in a single-patty hamburger with fixins.

Back to the hour-long walker: This person may have a resting metabolic rate of 1,750 and baseline activity-based energy usage of 875 calories. Without exercise, this person burned 2,625 calories. With an entire hour of daily exercise he is burning just 225 more. Hardly seems worth the effort if time is short and you do not love exercise.

So now that I've talked you out of the need for exercise. Let's talk about the benefits.

We've spent a lot of time in this book talking about the need to cycle your body through its portfolio of metabolic and biological states for correct physiological function. One of those states is going to be a state of intense physical exertion. Those of us who are truly sedentary don't naturally experience this state. This is why we blow up at our family, our kids, our spouses, or have emotional outbursts at work. It's the stress, tension and "toxins" that build up which we have not addressed with exercise. Our days of getting to "eat what we kill" are long gone, and we have not replaced the killing.

If you've ever gone through the process of considering breeds of dogs you might want to adopt, the discussion inevitably turns to "This breed needs room to run"; "This dog is a working dog"; "This dog is a herding dog, and will be depressed without the right outlets for energy". What happens to those dogs without the right environment is well known. Certain breeds get angry, exhibit anxiety behaviors, or act out. Working dogs without working challenges have behavioral problems. These dogs become hard to manage. Anger, depressions, misbehavior: Does it sound like some of the vents we may be using ourselves? Why would we give better consideration to the conditions for our pets than we give to our own activities and environment?

With that as an entrée, here are some of the observed benefits of exercise:

- Reduced depression
- Better sense of well-being
- Euphoria, optimism
- Better ability to relax
- Better health (joints, muscles, heart, inflammatory response)
- Better energy
- Ability to do and enjoy more challenging activities

- More physical desires and appetites, higher sexual appetite
- Better interpersonal skills (less stressed, better ability to engage in activities)
- ***Impact on Autophagy – cleaning out the body's metabolic waste and protecting against a host of diseases***
- ***Increased muscle hypertrophy and improved muscle response and tone***

As you read through this list – you will note that is pretty much nothing "science-sounding" except for the last two bullets on autophagy and muscle development – and the impact of these science bullets is not unrelated to the benefits articulated at the top of the list. While hundreds of observational studies have connected some or all of benefits listed above to exercise, the reason exercise has such a strong impact on sense of health, wellness, and desire to live life, is not completely understood.

We know that exercise improves mental health – just as in the example with working dogs – but we have not identified how exercise might be connected to the metabolism of brain chemicals that improve mental wellness. In fact, the US National Institutes of Health in June of 2015 launched a five year $170 M research program to better understand how the body changes in response to physical activity. It seems like this is science we should have already settled, but in fact, we have not. The aim of the NIH work is to better understand on a molecular level how exercise changes or improves tissues or organs with an obvious objective to understand the quality and kind of exercise that will create the greatest health benefit (Wang, 2015).

While I said that the scientific impact of exercise on overall health variables is not completely understood, lets discuss briefly a couple of generally accepted scientific conclusions on the impacts of exercise. The first known beneficial biological effect of exercise is an increase in autophagy. Recall in Chapter 5 that I discussed how short-term fasting also causes an increase in autophagy. Autophagy is the metabolic process by which the body destroys and digests old and broken cells and proteins. Autophagy is important **for** improving cellular and organ function and removing waste products from the body. Robust autophagy may also reduce the risk that malfunctioning cells become cancerous.   There is evidence the process of autophagy protects against neurodegenerative disorders, infections, inflammatory diseases, ageing and insulin resistance (C He, 2012). Defects in the autophagy process which lead to an accumulation of toxic proteins are a common denominator in both Alzheimer's and Parkinson's (Moussa, 2016).

An article published in the journal *Nature* in 2012 studied the impact of exercise on autophagy by producing genetically modified mice. Mice were modified so that the metabolic pathway that excites exercise-induced autophagy did not work.   By comparing these mice to normal mice in the presence of exercise, the authors were able to show that exercise induces autophagy, and that the mice with exercise-induced autophagy (the normal mice) had better endurance and better glucose metabolism than the modified mice. The research also suggests that the mechanism that drives exercise-induced autophagy is the same one that excites fasting-induced autophagy. Fasting and exercise are both drivers of metabolic clean up. Cellular clean-up may also contribute to the sense of well-being that comes after exercise as you purge those waste products from the body.

The other obvious (and well-established) benefit of exercise is muscle development. Strength training, which usually means lifting weights, contributes to muscle size and strength due to a process called **hypertrophy**, which is the process by which protein synthesis of muscle fibers occurs as a result of the stimulus and damage caused to muscle fibers by strength training. Exercise further improves the nerve impulses that recruit your muscles, and this contributes to improved *muscle tone*. Muscle tone is the taught-ness in muscles that come because they are in a state of readiness and partial state of contraction. Without proper muscle tone, muscles can look flabby. By activating the neurological circuits that recruit your muscles for great exertion under stress, strength training improves muscle tone in both men and women.

An article in the 2001 *International Journal on Sports Nutrition* established that exercise has a profound impact on muscle size and tone – but only if you supply your body ample amino acids (protein) during the 24 to 48 hour period after exercise. So remember, it is important if you are strength training that you use the rule of thumb to "eat your weight in grams of protein" (KD Tipton, 2001). (That means a weight trainer who weighs 150 pounds should target 150 grams of protein per day.) The profound impact that muscle development can have on your appearance and confidence cannot be understated for men or for women. If you are approaching your ideal weight – within 30 pounds – you may incorporate regular strength training into your exercise routine with a goal of achieving muscularity at the level of 3 to 4 based on the scale in **Table 3** of Chapter 2. You don't have to increase your hours spent exercising, but can rather replace some of the conditioning type exercise with strength training. High Intensity Interval Training programs ("HIIT"), which are today available everywhere you go, can also help you to build muscle mass without needing to "pump iron". We'll discuss how to incorporate HIIT and strength training into your weekly routine shortly.

EXERCISE AND YOUR LIFESTYLE.

One of the most common refrains you hear from people – especially parents – who have not engaged in structured exercise for a while is "There is no way I have time to exercise. My life is completely full with kids, activities, job, church, etc. etc. etc." For that reason I decided it was important to discuss exercise and your lifestyle for a few minutes, and seek to get you to think about how easy it is to fix your priorities.

Some of us may have engaged in sports or physical activities as children. Some of us may have continued exercise at least through some or all of adulthood, but somewhere along the way to job, and family if that's the case, you decided you were making a new commitment in life that would have to crowd out exercise, at least for the time being. Maybe you'd return to it later. The fact is that for you, later usually never happens.

So here is the plain reality: anyone who says they don't have time for exercise is full of bullshit. Sorry to say that, but it's a fact. If you are obese, I will ask you for 4 to 5 hours a week. If you are approaching your ideal weight, I'd ask you for as little as 25 minutes per day for 4 or 5 days a week – i.e. as little as 100 minutes. That's less than the length of a feature film. With your renewed energy from exercise, you might find you need at least 15 minutes less sleep every night (105 minutes per week). If your lost weight reduces sleep apnea, you'll save even more sleep. If you've read to here, you know that you are also going to free up some of the time you normally spend constantly feeding your gullet.

The fact is – and I know this sounds cliché (some things reach cliché status because they are true): what few things in life are more important than your health? It's all you got. As an example, you find a lot of families with kids become engrossed with the activities of their kids – and enter a rat race of driving them to activities and practices beyond the pale of reason. Could your child do one less activity, and you use that recovered time to more than cover your weekly exercise budget? Maybe pick the one that won't help him or her get into college or get that big scholarship, and kill that one. Or maybe you could go for a run during your kid's practice, rather than sitting there playing with your phone. Maybe you have no family. If you are young in a career maybe everyone in your office expects you to work til 10 PM. If that's the case, how about quietly jumping out for lunch and grabbing 40 minutes in the gym. You can eat at your desk. Or get up early and catch an hour before you show up. Sorry if this seems like tough love. If I could connect with you directly, I could help you figure out how to make this work in your current lifestyle, but it's probably something you can also figure out yourself.

Here's another fact: there is only one way to be successful with regular and reliable exercise: **you have to be selfish about it**. Otherwise you won't do it. Decide that this is something you are going to do for yourself and don't bend or compromise about it. Sneak in the gym before work (BTW - you don't have to join a gym). Duck out for lunch. You don't have to tell anybody what you are doing, but be honest if they ask. Find someone to drive your kid to practice and take turns. Your spouse knows you have to work late a couple nights a week – that can include the quick detour to exercise. By the way, you also need to support your spouse in the same endeavor.

Remember, **there is always something you could do that seems more selfless than exercise** – helping your spouse with dinner, extra time on an important project at the office, or helping your kids with their homework. If you set your priorities based on these alternatives, you will frankly never get something done that has the same level of importance as all those other things.

In the same vein, a lot of people drop off the exercise wagon after a life event. A marriage, starting a new job, having a first child. "I'm going to be too busy with the new kid." These are the critical times when it is most important to maintain consistency, not shed it. Don't skip even a day of your routine if you can avoid it. If you're in the hospital with a new baby, say to the spouse "Honey, you ok if I run out for a couple hours and I'll be back with dinner?" (I'm sure there is also some reasonable analogy for the reverse genders as well.) That way you establish for the spouse and for yourself that despite the new addition to the family, you will remain committed to this critical health requirement. Getting back to it "someday" means not for a very long time if ever.

Here's the irony of the "I have no time" argument: You are going to find that when you exercise, even with minimal exercise, you are going to feel more energy, more *desire for activity*, and more eagerness to attack life and its challenges. All that low energy and lassitude you've been feeling, that you have attributed to "I'm getting a little older," is actually the torpor of inactivity weighing you down. I know a police officer who is 53 and plays ice hockey three nights a week – he has so much energy that he can skate up and down the ice like everyone else is standing still. He attributes his energy to his activity. It's an autocatalytic effect. Remember all those times at work that you had that afternoon dip in productivity? You fucked around and did nearly nothing between 2 and 4 PM? If you had stopped for exercise before work, or jumped out at lunch, that rarely would happen. You just spent one of your two void hours, and gained the other back in productivity. If you exercise, your energy will drive you to attack and do more faster, it will make you more productive. So that 2 to 4 hours of weekly exercise will buy you 10 hours in increased output.

Time spent in exercise. As I mentioned in the intro, you don't need to spend a lot of time exercising. It's more important that you reach high intensity for a few minutes during each session of exercise. Five to fifteen minutes at high intensity can be enough. I suggest the most time in exercise for the newly committed weight losers (still not a lot of time, unless you want to spend a lot of time). You need to send new signals that will activate your metabolism and gradually develop intensity. As we'll discuss, if you are very fat, you should shoot for an hour per day 4 to 5 days per week. As you develop, you should focus on high-intensity interval training that can last as little as 25 minutes as long as it includes 5 to 15 minutes at high intensity. If you plan to engage in strength training as you near your ideal weight, then you will need to maintain 45 minutes to an hour at least three days per week.

Golfer Padraig Harrrington won three major PGA tournaments between 2006 and 2008, and rose as high as No. 3 in PGA world rankings. Six years later, at the age of 43 he was practically unranked and forgotten. In November 2015, he was ranked 385 and lost his PGA status, but the following March, he entered the Honda Classic and won, capturing his first PGA Major in over six year. His secret: doing less: "When I was a kid on tour, I'd work out every night, doing 90 minutes of cardio and 60 minutes of weights." Today, according to Harrington, he invests no more than 10 minutes per day on cardio and 20 on weights. He says that this short intense burst activates his endorphins and leaves him craving exercise for the next day (Murphy, 2015). You will find this if you reach high intensity in your daily exercise: craving that euphoria for the next day.

An article in *The Wall Street Journal* entitled "Why Everything You Know About Aging Is Probably Wrong", included "Myth No. 6: More Exercise is Better". A growing number of studies suggest that more exercise isn't always better.

> "You get to a point of diminishing returns," says James O'Keefe, a professor of medicine at the University of Missouri-Kansas City. In a study to be published this month, Dr. O'Keefe, and co-authors tracked 1,098 joggers and 3,950 non-joggers from 2001 to 2013; all were part of the Copenhagen City Heart Study, under way since 1976. Overall, the runners in the Copenhagen study lived longer than the non-runners: 6.2 years longer for the men and 5.6 years longer for the women. But the new study discovered that those who ran more than four hours a week at a fast pace – of 7 miles per hour or more – **lost** much, if not all, of the longevity benefits. The group that saw the biggest improvements … jogged from one to 2.4 hours weekly at 5 to 7 mph and took at least two days off from vigorous exercise per week. Other studies have come to similar conclusions … In research published this year, … the death rate for runners is 30% to 45% below that for non-runners. But the mortality benefits were similar for all runners, even those who ran ***five to 10 minutes per day*** (Tergesen, 2014) [emphasis supplied].

Bottom line, allow an hour at least 4 days a week if you are obese, otherwise, allow 25 minutes per day for high intensity days, and 45 minutes to an hour on strength training days

Working exercise into your lifestyle. There are actually only a few possible formats in our American lifestyle and culture that you can drive an exercise routine.

If you are a **professional student** or **house maker**, you typically have opportunities to get your exercise because you have more control over your schedule. If you're a college student, you can do it before or after classes (I realize students rarely get up early), at dinner time, or in the evening. If you are a house maker, you typically have a good deal of flexibility during the day, even if you have kids: there are windows when they are at school, camps, or activities. Very young kids should be in day care at least a couple have days a week so you get those windows. What I'm saying is there are never any excuses unless you invent them yourselves. If you are in one of these roles where there is typically more flexibility, it is important that you ***establish a routine*** that is consistent and repetitious for when you exercise. Flexibility can be a bane if you say "I'll have plenty of opportunities to squeeze a workout in." Remember, you need 4 or 5 sessions a week, and if you make it ok to put it off, you'll end up not doing it.

If you are a **working stiff**, you have three options: go get your exercise before work, slip out at lunch during work, or do it after work. Any of these options are A-OK. If you do physical labor or shift work, you may not be able to slip out for lunch. But in the same vein, depending on the labor (for example if you carry bricks), you may not need additional exercise. If you are in doubt, you should incorporate it. Remember it's not just time, but intensity that matters. If you are seated and fastening nuts on bolts in a factory you may not meet any reasonable standard for intensity.

If you are a **working stiff with kids and family**, it's really difficult to stop for exercise after work. You can't leave work too early, and if you exercise after work, you'll often get home too late. Plus it's an unfair reality of the American workplace that if you get to the office at 6 AM and leave at 4 PM, you just worked an hour more than your colleagues, but you are "the guy that leaves work at 4". Better to get up and stop on the way to work, or slip out at lunch to give you an afternoon boost. If you plan to exercise at home after kids are in bed, it can be done, but you'll often find you feel too tired by the time you are free.

As we'll discuss shortly, the **internet** has been a great liberator allowing you to work out very effectively at home. That being said, I do recommend you join a gym. It will increase your variety of workout and opportunity, and your sense of commitment to a new lifestyle. You also probably drive by one every day on your way to work, or school, or in your regular travels, so it only involves 5 minutes additional investment to pull in and pull out. With at least two anchors in your week at a gym or fitness facility, you will feel more invested, more like you need to get value from your investment, and more likely to treat exercise as a legitimate personal obligation rather than an optional activity. Some people will use web-based inspiration for days they travel for work or have to be at home, but use a professional gym days they work in the office. You'll conclude what works best for you, but my recommendation is you start an exercise commitment with a professional gym four to five days per week, and move to web-based exercise for day's you'd otherwise miss ... and then only after you've developed some sense of routine and personal commitment.

Key success factors for working exercise into your lifestyle. Whatever your place in life's journey and whatever your family obligations, here is what I would insist is necessary for lifestyle success:

Find a pattern. You absolutely will not stay on an exercise program if you have to figure out every day or every week when you are going to get to your workout. People who are successful with exercise always follow a pattern. Your goal should be for five days a week and give yourself two days off (unless you love exercise). You could hit mornings on the way to work 5 days, or do that 3 days and take a run at lunchtime twice. I like to take my weekends off, but you might like to hit the gym Tuesday and Thursday, do a web-based routine when you work from home one day a week, and then work out Saturday and Sunday. There are hundreds of patterns that you can contrive and enjoy, that don't have to make you feel like you have a second job, or are stealing time from family.

Give yourself 2 consecutive days off. Give yourselves 2 consecutive days off per week. For most of you, especially with families, this makes the most sense two do on weekends, but it doesn't have to be weekends. The days off give you motivation, inspiration, and a needed break, especially if you do not love exercise. It also prevents you from getting something called "exercise fatigue" or "overtraining", a phenomenon that can cause fatigue, listlessness, and poor workouts because your body does not have time to recover. (This phenomenon mostly affects people who are engaged in high intensity strength training.) If you find yourself starting to enjoy exercise and you find yourself becoming an exercise addict, it's ok to exercise six days per week, but absolutely give yourself one full recovery day every week.

Allow yourself a flex day. The first lifestyle principal here was to find a pattern. That pattern should incorporate five planned exercise days per week. In your mind, you should know that if you have an important family obligation, a big presentation at work, or an unplanned business trip, and recognizing this stuff comes up every week, it's ok to skip one workout a week. The psychology of knowing that it is ok to do this will reduce stress and allow you to feel you can be better committed to your planned routine. If your sessions end up averaging four days per week, plan to have at least two of those be full hour sessions. You'll get plenty of exercise time that way. If you have to miss more than two days due to "emergencies" force yourself to reschedule one. Don't cheat. Otherwise you'll end up on a treadmill of rationalization and not one of exercise. I find that most people have less anxiety knowing they can skip once per week if they are in the weeds, but that most don't actually end up using this out very often after they've established a strong routine.

This section was written to motivate you about the idea that you can fit exercise into your lifestyle without major sacrifice. If you haven't performed structured exercise in many years, or possibly ever, the next two sections are meant to get you started on how to jump in with a very low barrier to entry.

EXERCISE MODALITIES – WHAT'S IN THE ARSENAL?

For purposes of this book and most fitness literature, there are really just three kinds of exercise: **conditioning, strength training, and stretching**. Let me define these in reverse order.

Stretching means extending and cycling your muscles and ligaments, and also articulating your joints and skeletal elements, often in preparation for other exercise. In this context stretching extends muscles and tendons, increases blood flow to muscles and better prepares you for other exercise by creating a state of readiness and stability in muscles. This makes subsequent exercise safer and more effective. Stretching is not only appropriate as preparation for other exercise. Yoga exercise focuses primarily on stretching and articulating muscles and skeleton as a standalone method of exercise. Yoga improves not only muscle conditioning, but also functional strength, balance, and body mechanics. (In the context of exercise, functional strength means the ability to recruit muscles effectively and use muscles and skeletal elements with confidence and coordination in order to perform actions that (1) require strength and balance and (2) are actually useful in real life. "Pumping iron" to be able to perform the same isolated movement with a very heavy weight would be kind of the opposite of functional strength.) If you enjoy yoga, you can mix it in on one of your weekly exercise days as you move towards your ideal weight.

Strength Training means pursuing the objective of increasing muscle size, mass, and strength. Strength training involves the free-weights and muscle-isolating machines you see at most gyms and fitness clubs. Most personal training sessions have historically been focused on strength training. Persons approaching ideal weight may decide to incorporate strength training in the exercise program. It allows you to improve strength, replace lost fat with muscle, reduce osteoporosis,and improves the aesthetics of your body. Strength training is not as important in the early part of a weight loss regimen if you are significantly overweight. So if you are more than 20% above your ideal weight, you can hold off on strength training until you are about 15- to 20% above your objective.

Conditioning usually means focusing on your fitness, endurance, and stamina. The most prominent element of conditioning is aerobic fitness. Typically cycling your heart rate to a high level to improve heart health, endurance, stamina, circulation, and to drive those metabolic states that will contribute to health and wellness. When I discuss shortly the importance of reaching a level of intensity in exercise, the goal will be articulated in terms of your heart rate. Conditioning work used to be called "aerobic exercise" (involves heavy breathing of oxygen) or "cardio" (involves heart), and I'll use these terms interchangeably, but they are becoming a little bit dated in the exercise community. Conditioning also includes developing the skills you need to perform life and athletic activities. That means training to improve your recruitment of "fast-twitch" muscles for bursts of movements, improving balance and agility, and developing and training the body mechanics needed to perform optimal movement in sports activities such as sprinting or batting a baseball. Most of these elements of conditioning will be available to you naturally in the context of performing "HIIT" exercise as discussed in the next paragraph.

HIIT is the acronym for "High Intensity Interval Training". This generic term is fairly broad, but always describes exercise in which you engage in rapid bursts of all-out 102% effort followed by brief periods of rest. For example, 20 seconds of burpees, followed by 20 seconds of mountain climbers, followed by 20 percent of rest. Even the rest periods are sometimes active – jogging in place for example. HIIT programs are generally only 20 to 30 minutes, but they will wear you out in this short time. HIIT doesn't fall into one of the three categories above because it combines always at least two of them: strength training and conditioning. Some HIIT routines also incorporate yoga moves, so these also include stretching. This type of exercise is one of the most time efficient you can engage, because you are performing exercise that improves your conditioning and endurance, but also improving your strength. Good programs are organized to mix modes and intensity so that not a single second is wasted.

There are many **HIIT** programs and routines available on the internet. Some of the most popular programs you hear about all the time are HIIT programs. These include **Tabata** routines, which usually consists of 8 rounds of intense exercise punctuated by 20 seconds of rest. It also includes functional routines with novel equipment like **kettlebell** routines. The famous **P90X** program is a HIIT routine even though its sponsors may take exception to that characterization or note certain differences. P90X programs are laser focused on reducing body fat and increasing muscle mass and tone in order to improve your appearance. The focus on muscularity means P90X routines may pull in some novel equipment like bands or bars, but overall equipment needed is minimal. In the same vein, **CrossFit**, is a tremendously popular HIIT modality taking off in specialized gyms all over the US. CrossFit today includes many dozens of different kinds of worthwhile workouts, but with a focus on fitness and muscle development. Core CrossFit routines incorporate high intensity movements for aerobic fitness and strength. You will see folks in CrossFit gyms who look like they have focused on dedicated body building but have gained their size and muscularity solely via CrossFit group classes. CrossFit routines do tend to use a lot of specialized equipment for strength elements (kettlebells, barbells, dumbbells, bands, etc.) so that it is significantly restricted to specialized CrossFit gyms around the US and the rest of the world.

So do you need to go to a gym? On the correct venue for exercise the internet has been a great liberator. There are thousands of great exercise videos and programs on the web that you can do in your house with either no equipment or a couple of light dumbbells, including HIIT workouts. Many of these programs are fantastic. At-home routines are not easy light-weight exercise for bored house-makers. They are not routines that echo the Jane Fonda jazzercise videos of the 1980's. These are the real deal and they can kick your ass. All you need is a computer or internet-connected TV and some space to work.

Here are a few great examples:

HASFIT (hasfit.com) – Coach Joshua Kozak and his wife Claudia have posted hundreds of free workouts for strength (organized by muscle group), endurance and cardio (high intensity workouts). Many of the home workouts require no equipment at all, and some require a set of light dumbells which you can buy at Amazon or Target, or at any discount or sporting good store. Beware, an advanced workout will take you down in just 20 minutes.

Scott Herman Fitness (muscularstrength.com) – Scott Herman is focused on muscularity and bodybuilding. He has many great routines that will elevate your approach to strength training if you are in this phase of your exercise evolution. If you are in the gym doing strength training, an hour workout should include at least 15 minutes of a cardio activity that will reach high intensity, as discussed shortly in this chapter.

PopSugar Fitness (www.popsugar.com/workouts) – PopSugar has a great portfolio of workouts very well organized around cardio, strength training, yoga, and beginner. While these workouts are oriented towards women's exercise, the advanced ones would easily kick the asses of many men. A great resource of workouts of all modalities, and a variety of focused body parts and exercise durations.

All three of these properties have both destination sites (listed above in parentheses) and YouTube channels. There are many more great sites and individuals posting great programs, so this was just intended to get you started (and not to endorse these over others not mentioned). In some ways programs like P90X started the trend to high intensity interval training, but these are paid programs with DVD's and books. I hope the creator of P90X, Tony Horton, made many millions. Unfortunately for his business, today you do not need to reach into your wallets for great instruction

Now that I have given my mini-advertisement for YouTube based fitness programs I'll remind you that I believe **joining** a gym or fitness facility and **exercising there** at least two days a week is something that is important and worthwhile. It enables you to use equipment you won't have access to at home, to overcome the intimidation if you are not comfortable in a gym, to potentially meet trainers or others who could teach and inspire you, to try a variety of exercise modalities in fitness classes – and most importantly, to feel you've made a hard commitment that is part of a fixed established routine.

If you are self-conscious due to your weight, just go right up to the treadmill when you get to the gym. It's easy to figure out and non-threatening. Or ask the club to arrange a screening with a trainer. The trainer can get you started in a non-intimidating way, and you can reduce your paid sessions after a couple of months. If you feel like people are judging you because you are fat, the reality is that those crazy fit people are at worst thinking "She's a wreck, but she's here showing up to make herself better." And so people generally want to help you. Judgment is reserved for people who didn't show up in the first place.

A Personal Exercise Modality --- or "What Do I Do to Exercise?"

The answer to how you should exercise depends on where you are with your weight. Below I'm going to propose you consider three configurations depending on how many pounds you have exceeding your ideal weight. This simple evolutionary prescription is based on the objective of providing you a course of action using structured exercise time of 4 to 5 times per week. If you find yourself really enjoying doing more exercise, you may do more structured exercise. You'll almost certainly find yourself enjoying more active non-structured exercise as you find more energy (hiking, playing outdoor games, pool time, etc.).

You should get a few key messages from **Table 13**. First, if you are **obese** or very obese, you simply need to get moving. Don't seek high levels of intense continuous exertion, just an hour of walking – and you should seek to do that five days a week. You will start to restore the physiological and metabolic pathways that are driven by activity. I suggest you do it on a treadmill in the gym. If you are very overweight, again, walking in and walking straight to that treadmill is one of the least intimidating exercise evolutions you can make in a public setting. Those ultra fit people you will also see in the gym – some of them used to look like you – and most of them would appreciate the opportunity to help and encourage you. There is fraternity in what you are doing.

As I said, **for the obese**, get on a treadmill and walk; however, I am going to ask you to reach a **high intensity zone** for at least a two to five minutes during each session evolving to 10 minutes. *We'll talk about what high intensity means shortly.* As you get more comfortable, in addition to the high intensity period, you should spend an increasing part of the hour in a jog or run instead of walking.

If you are not obese but you are **significantly overweight** (say 40 to 70 pounds over ideal weight), I'll ask you to maintain some plain walking and jogging in a couple of sessions per week, but with a longer interval of intense exertion and running during the hour. I'll also ask you to mix in some **HIIT training**. HIIT can be done easily in a fitness class at the gym, or with any of the many excellent online videos. You can pick shorter workouts with online video by selecting around 25 minutes of work. If you take two days walking / running and two days on structured HIIT exercise, you can use the last day to pick your preferred modality: another day of walking / running, another HIIT session focusing on an area of interest (abs, arms, glutes), or a day of stretching / yoga. If you pick yoga, I recommend you also spend 15 minutes of intense conditioning (treadmill, stationary bike, etc.) before your class. *I will talk more about the importance of "HIIT training" shortly.*

If you are merely **overweight** but have moved within 30 to 40 pounds of your ideal weight, it's ok to start to blend in some dedicated strength training as shown in the table, especially for men. This is an easy way to start to substitute some muscle mass for fat, and increase your "allowable" ideal weight per Table 5 by increasing your muscularity. For women who don't want "massive" muscle, strength training at reasonable levels of weight will improve your shape and muscle tone. If you have low muscle mass and tone, adding mass will happen very quickly if you fall into level 1 or 2 muscularity of Table 3. *I will talk more about the nature of strength training shortly.*

	Day 1	Day 2	Day 3	Day 4	Day 5
Obese *or 70 to 100 lb +* *over ideal weight*	one hour on treadmill, with 5 to 15 minutes of **intense** exertion	one hour on treadmill, with 5 to 15 minutes of **intense** exertion	one hour on treadmill, with 5 to 15 minutes of **intense** exertion	one hour on treadmill, with 5 to 15 minutes of **intense** exertion	one hour on treadmill, with 5 to 15 minutes of **intense** exertion
Significantly Overweight *or 40 to 70 lb* *over ideal weight*	one hour on treadmill, with 15 to 20 minutes of **intense** exertion	**HIIT training** - either group **fitness class** or **online video**, 25 to 50 minutes	15 minutes **conditioning**, with at least 5 minutes **intense exertion** **Your Day** - 25 to 50 minutes yoga, HIIT, strength training, what you enjoy	**HIIT training** - either group **fitness class** or **online video**, 25 to 50 minutes	one hour on treadmill, with 15 to 20 minutes of **intense** exertion
Overweight *less than ~30 to 40 lb* *over ideal weight*	**HIIT training** - either group **fitness class** or **online video**, 25 to 50 minutes	--- 15 minutes **conditioning**, at least 5 minutes **intense**, --- 5 to 10 minutes stretching or balance **Strength Training** for 30 to 45 minutes	**HIIT training** - either group **fitness class** or **online video**, 25 to 50 minutes	--- 15 minutes **conditioning**, at least 5 minutes **intense**, --- 5 to 10 minutes stretching or balance **Strength Training** for 30 to 45 minutes	15 minutes **conditioning**, with at least 5 minutes **intense exertion** **Your Day** - 25 to 50 minutes yoga, HIIT, strength training, what you enjoy

Table 13 – Exercise modality based on excess weight.

High Intensity Zone conditioning goes to getting your heart rate high, your circulation high, and your metabolic energy recruitment high. It is this kind of metabolic turnover related to exercise that will help you excite the enhanced level of overall energy and the ability of your body to reach exercise-induced autophagy and euphoria I discussed earlier in this chapter. For this reason, I recommended that even if you are obese or very obese, you reach a level of high intensity for at least a minute or two even from your first workout. What this means is that if you are doing one hour of treadmill, you pick a five minute block where you will crank up the equipment. High intensity will mean that your heart rate is between 65 and 85 percent of your maximum heart rate. Your maximum heart rate is the maximum rate you should reach during exercise for purposes of cardiac safety. The rule of thumb for calculating maximum heart rate is "220 minus your age". There are other sources that propose more refined equations based on more detailed clinical data, and some sources say that this method can understate your correct maximum for older persons, but the simple formula is usually close, it's a great rule of thumb and easy to remember.

$$Maximum\ Heart\ Rate = 220 - Your\ Age \qquad (Eqn.\ 9)$$

$$Bottom\ of\ Intense\ Zone = 0.65*(220 - Your\ Age) \qquad (Eqn.\ 10)$$

$$Top\ of\ Intense\ Zone = 0.85*(220 - Your\ Age) \qquad (Eqn.\ 11)$$

The first equation calculates your maximum safe heart rate based on your age. Use the second equation to calculate your 65% level and the second equation to calculate your 85% level.

Example – Bob is 43. Using (Eqn. 9) he calculates that his maximum heart rate should be 220 – 43 = 177 beats per minute. His exercise level in the intense training zone starts at 65% of his maximum, or 0.65 x 177 = 115 beats per minute. The top of his intense training range is 85% of his maximum or 0.85 x 177 = 151 beats per minute.

Many treadmills and other conditioning machines will give you a target based on your input age and exertion level, and almost all modern conditioning machines will calculate your heart rate. You can use the above equations to estimate your range a single time and use that information to evaluate your heart rate during your exercise.

What I you need to do with your hour of walking is to start increase the pace on the treadmill to between 5.5 and 8.5 miles per hour so that you are in a run and hold it for as long as you can – up to a maximum of 5 minutes. Over time, you will increase your pace to a little bit in that 5.5 to 8.5 mph range, and also increase your time. Increase either the pace or time a little bit every few sessions. Your goal should be to hold your high intensity zone for 5 to 7 minutes by the end of 12 weeks. If you are able to monitor your heart rate during your exercise – seek to get your heart rate above 80% of max for at least one to two of those minutes. For the rest of your hour, you can maintain that rapid walk or jog. The low intensity part of your workout should also increase over time from walking to jogging/running for most of that hour. Again, this will ensure that your body has no doubt that it exercised, and it will drive the metabolic cycling and exercise-induced autophagy that you need.

HIIT training in your routine. As I mentioned earlier, "HIIT" stands for high-intensity interval training. It's a broad term that is sometimes used on its own, but also can be used to describe very popular exercise programs such as P90X CrossFit, and kettle-ball workouts. There used to be a sense that exercise was either "aerobic" or "strength" training. Persons dedicated to HIIT training combine aerobic and strength training into a single modality of exercise. The long term trend in the fitness universe weighs heavily in favor of HIIT. If you go to a commercial gym the facility can help you pick classes that fit this model, or you can choose a CrossFit gym. If you prefer to do HIIT exercise at home, you can purchase a P90X program or use any of hundreds of free online videos. Specific programs may rise and fall in popularity, but the concept and value of HIIT is not going away. Machines in gyms often aim to isolate particular muscle groups, so that you have to combine many exercises to reach your entire body.

HIIT training incorporates movements that support functional strength: compound movements that recruit related muscles and enable you to improve not only muscle size, but functional strength, your balance, coordination, and ability to use your strength in real-world activities. These types of programs combine aerobic conditioning seamlessly with strength movements so that you get a great aerobic challenge, an element of exercise essential for autophagy but often overlooked in the gym. Combining conditioning and strength challenges also ensures that you get very high density of benefit from the time you spend in exercise. You may consider dedicated strength training optional if you enjoy HIIT type training and are getting 4 or 5 sessions per week. You can see that some of the CrossFit adherents have some of the best fitness, muscularity, and shape in the world, and don't engage in dedicated strength training.

Strength training will involve machines and free weights you see in the gym. If you feel intimidated by this equipment, hire a personal training for one session per week to get you started. There are also many programs and videos online that you can use to teach yourself (including HASFIT and Scott Herman). This book is not an exercise manual. My goal is to inspire and motivate you to do what you need to do, and not waste ink on detailed programs readily available online. Note that strength training is not a mandatory element of your exercise program. It's ok to maintain HIIT type program if that is what you enjoy.

Ensure that you maintain 4 to 5 sessions per week of dedicated exercise and you always focus on increase your dedication and intensity as your strength and fitness improves. Don't get in a rut. With strength training, you can add muscle size and mass very quickly if you fall in the categories of Level 1 or Level 2 of Table 3 in particular. You will see results within 12 weeks. If you are strength training, engage in at least 2 sessions of 30 to 50 minutes per week, and you can do up to 5 sessions. Just make sure if you are doing 5 sessions, that you include at least 15 minutes of aerobic conditioning either before or after these strength workouts in which you reach at least 80% of your aerobic maximum from the MHR equations and maintain that for at least 5 minutes (i.e. you want to approach the top of that 65- to 86% range). Also, simply eat your ideal weight in grams of protein every day and you will gain mass fairly quickly if you are a man, and tone and definition fairly quickly if you are a woman. A person whose ideal weight is 150 lbs. needs to eat 150 grams of protein per day. Prepackaged protein shakes, beef jerky, and canned fish are great ways to hit that target quickly.

EXERCISE - CONCLUSIONS

Exercise is indispensable if you plan to reach your ideal weight. There are a number of reasons for this. First exercise is essential if you seek to feel healthy, optimistic, and in order to develop the energy and determination you need to reach your ideal weight.

Exercise cycles your metabolism and is shown scientifically to induce autophagy, the process by which your body identifies, destroys, and disposes of old cells and malfunctioning proteins. This increases health and well-being, and reduces the risk of cancer and other diseases. You'll feel more optimism and less depression.

When you exercise, it is essential that you reach a period of high intensity (the high intensity zone). If you've ever done any intense aerobic exercise, this is the level of exertion where you are "sucking wind" and wondering how long you can sustain. If you are a beginner to exercise, you only need to reach that type of intensity for 2 to 5 minutes. You may increase that some as you gain experience, but 7 to 10 minutes are plenty. That high intensity is needed to "exercise your metabolism" and drive you into those metabolic states that induce well-being and metabolic recover.

You don't need to exercise a lot. You can aim for 3 to 5 hours a week in 4 or 5 workouts. If you are obese you should allow an hour, but spend most of it at a rapid walk. Don't forget to reach high intensity for 2 to 5 minutes and then gradually increase it by a few minutes.

After you reach a level within around 70 pounds of ideal weight, you can start to blend in some HIIT workouts. You will find many such workouts online, and they also include well-known programs online or paid programs like CrossFit and P90x. Many classes in gyms fall into this category as well. Good HIIT exercise programs only last 20 to 30 minutes, so when you reach this stage of development, you can spend a few days a week with a really quick exercise regime. After a HIIT workout, you may decide to add 10 or 15 minutes of regular cardio, balance, or stretching to round out an hour.

If you reach the neighborhood of 30 pounds above your ideal weight, you may decide to incorporate pure strength training, especially if you are male. Keep in mind that great HIIT programs do a great job of developing muscle, overall body strength, conditioning, and aesthetics, so that isolated strength training isn't absolutely essential. If you do include direct strength training, you can add muscle mass quickly. Remember to eat your weight in protein grams every day while strength training. Also, take 15 minutes to do some traditional cardio and ensure that you hit that high intensity window of 65- to 85% of your maximum heart rate and hold it for at least 5 minutes.

Remember that exercise is **essential** for success. Assertions that your lifestyle can't include it are nothing but excuses. Having the energy of fitness will save you more time than you invest. Exercise is fundamental for you to condition your metabolism, and facilitate the energy, sense of well-being, and optimism you need to lose weight. The end result is that you are healthier, and you feel better, more energetic and more prepared to attack every challenge that comes from life.

Exercises – Chapter 7 Exercise

You're more likely to start and maintain exercise if you write down your plan.

1. Do you exercise 4 or 5 days a week now. If not, write down an plan that you think you could execute to find 45 minutes 5 days a week to sneak away and get real exercise. I need you to write down this plan even if you think it is largely impossible.

2. If you exercise now, list the three days, routines, or individual exercises you enjoy the most. If you don't exercise now, list three things you think you could enjoy in exercise.

1.

2.

3.

3. Write down a plan similar to Table 13 of what you'd like to do each day on a five-day routine. It doesn't have to be highly specific, but give yourself some hard days, and give yourself some variety.

Day 1	Day 2	Day 3	Day 4	Day 5

Chapter 8 – Holism: Putting it All Together

Reaching and maintaining your ideal weight takes rhythm. You probably thought I would say "discipline". Rhythm means getting comfortable with a set of patterns that enable your success. You will learn to identify and reinforce these patterns in this chapter and through a little bit of experience. Every other diet and fitness book \ will tell you exactly what to do. Exactly what to eat. "Just follow this set of steps and …" "Drink these milkshakes and ….", etc.

The problem with this approach is that it is usually about creating either a pattern of false promises, or a set of steps too specific and complex for you to adhere to indefinitely. It is very difficult to follow and maintain someone else's prescription, especially when it involves a lot of very specific steps around food and diet. Attrition is huge and benefits are marginal, especially considering that food quantity measured in calories is the only meaningful impactor of weight. My aim in this book has been to provide you principals, signposts, and guidance that will motivate you and ensure you succeed on terms you can develop and maintain.

> **EXERCISE PREVIEW**: UNCOVER YOUR PERSONAL FACTORS OF A WEEKLY RHYTHM. THINK ABOUT WHEN YOU ARE STRESSED, WHEN YOU TEND TO OVEREAT, WHEN YOU CAN GET WORKOUTS IN.

Reaching your ideal weight means eating fewer calories than you burn. You might create a deficit of 500 calories per day to lose weight. **Maintaining** your ideal weight means eating the same calories as you burn. The difference between "reaching" and "maintaining" isn't that great. It may be a sandwich per day, or a yogurt and a packet of trail mix. Some people might see this as a bad thing ("I have to diet for the rest of my life?"), but it's actually a huge benefit. Folks who take the mentality that "once I reach my goal, I can return to normal" only ensure that they will become fat again. Folks who find a rhythm of balance enjoy a permanent new lifestyle that has them feeling better and ***enjoying food more***.

In this final chapter, I am going to talk about the importance of developing patterns that are success-oriented but also fit your lifestyle, about identifying and managing rewards, about weighing yourself frequently, and about how to incorporate the concepts of hunger, fasting, nutrition, and exercise in establishing that rhythm for success. Finally, I will talk about success of others – what has worked for persons who lost a great deal of weight and kept it off for over 5 years. You'll learn that there is not one formula for success, but once you establish **your own** rhythm, you can develop and sustain permanent success.

REWARDS

Food is a reward. It should be viewed and enjoyed like a reward. Food is also a necessity. We need to eat nearly every day. Those of us who are overweight tend to overemphasize the reward aspect of eating (to the point that it becomes not very meaningful), and we ultimately fail to separate reward from necessity. Constant rewards make us fat and fatuous. In order to maintain an ideal weight, it is necessary to **identify and ration** food rewards. This sounds at the outset like it sucks, but the reality is that since we live in a society that provides a river of food, reward management actually makes eating better and more fulfilling.

There are two ways this can happen, and either way may be fine for you. First, if your reward rationing involves improving your diet, you may pretty quickly lose your appetite for cake and cinnamon buns and enjoy the foods you eat on a daily basis. Second, if you make your rewards special and correctly rationed, you'll appreciate those rewards more, and enjoy even better French Fries, or a bacon burger, than you do when you eat it for lunch every single day.

In our "river of food" world, we see these rewards coming at us constantly. You see examples everywhere in our culture. An executive I work with likes to reward a hard day's work for himself and his colleagues with a big meal at a restaurant of his choice every night. We are talking about nice restaurants with great food. Usually we have appetizers, salads, entrees, often desert. Along with this goes at least a couple of bottles of wine. If you add these meals up, you are passing 2,000 calories in a single meal. Ouch. A great meal for an occasional huge business victory or special occasion. For "Todd", it's rewarding a hard day's work. The problem is that we work hard every day, and you can't eat a 2,000 calorie dinner every night without getting fat (which Todd has done).

For those of us with families, we see rewards around children's activities constantly. This sounds horribly cliché to write, but "when I was a kid", we played soccer, we got some orange slices to rehydrate us. Today, kids get juice boxes and a bag of cookies. That's a treat.   Kid's birthday at school?   Cupcakes every week.   Halloween, Thanksgiving, Christmas? Parties at school. Candy inside eggs and ice cream after the hunt. Great victory in a sports game? Ice Cream after. Tough loss in a sports game? Ice Cream for consolation. Valentine's Day? Today kids come home with cards and candy. End of school party, end of camp party, end of lessons party, end of season party, end of class – all horrible food rewards every week or multiple times per week. It's a fact that these days, every children's activity is punctuated with a food reward. With the trend for kids towards organized activities, and the trend for constant food rewards, we end up with these types of food reward events 4, 5, maybe 6 or more times a week.

The same thing is happening to you at work. One of these parents buys too much candy or cupcakes or other treats for the kids event – where does it end up? Left out at work. And around 10:30 AM, we all eat it.

Or maybe you're are a manager at your job, and as part of morale and connectivity, you take your an employees out to lunch 3 or 4 days per week. Those burgers, chicken sandwiches with cheese and bacon, french fries, many of those plates have nearly a full-day's supply of calories.

So how do I define rewards? Well again in the veins of empowerment around "*On Friday's We Fast*", you need to identify and define your rewards yourself. You deserve three or four rewards per week. That works out to about every other day, and that should be plenty to keep you motivated. Let me give you a few examples.

- Sarah loves fast food breakfast – McDonalds, Burger King, Dunkin Donuts --- doesn't matter. A biscuit with eggs and bacon and some hash browns is heaven. She used to go there 2 or 3 times a week after the gym: whenever she had time before work. Shit, why shouldn't she? She just went to the gym. Then she realized her rewards were making her fat, so she decided that Wednesdays would be her McDonalds day. After all, its hump day. She **defined** the day and the reward, rather than leaving it open-ended. Now she doesn't have to have this internal guilty debate every morning on whether I should stop for food. The result of this change is that she **appreciate and enjoys** her McDonalds breakfast much more now that she gets to look forward to it every Wednesday.

- John's church has donuts every Sunday. A delicious sugar bomb that I could probably eat in a single bite – and then grab a second. It's a great reward, and after all, he deserves it because he made it to church. God wants to reward him. Unfortunately, its 20% of a day's calories that he couldn't afford to spend in 5 seconds once a week. So now he's decided that the last Sunday of the month is "Donut Sunday". On that day, if he's in the mood, he grab a donut and eats it without guilt. That donut tastes much better than when he sucks it down every week.

- Terry love to eat dinner in restaurants. When he goes he want to feel it's special. Appetizers and desert are often incorporated. It's a treat to himself and he doesn't want to worry about calories and healthiness. He used to find myself in restaurants 3 or 4 nights a week. Now he's decided that Saturday is "restaurant night". He takes the family and they do what they want: order whatever they want; the difference is that since this is not happening several times a week, or "whenever" and it has become a special occasion. If he needs to have dinner with clients for work, he eats a decent salad.

- Bill likes a stiff glass of whiskey before bed; however, often that whiskey was ending up being two tall whiskeys. When he did the math, he realized it was totaling about 2,400 calories a week. That's like an eighth day of eating! No wonder he was gaining weight. Now he still enjoys his whiskey, but limits it to either Thursday or Friday, and also Saturday night. Now he has a nice tall one and sometimes a second, but he's only using 600 calories for the week.

- Jane's company supplies free lunch for employees. She knows she shouldn't do it, but she just loves the pizza, burgers, and pasta that they serve and gravitates to it every day. She found herself getting fatter and fatter, until she realized just because it's free, she doesn't have to "get my money's worth" every single day. She was on the path to killing herself on the sword of obesity over a free lunch. She decided that Tuesdays are her unrestricted lunch day. She eats whatever she wants on Tuesdays, and the rest of the week, she eats her lunch off the salad bar with an ounce dressing.

- My wife and I like to unwind with half an hour of TV before we go to bed. We used to grab a snack every night – nachos, ice cream, whatever was around. You aren't expected to eat healthy after 10 PM. The problem was that both of us were gaining weight at a steady pace. We decided that Tuesdays were healthy snack night – usually hummus, and Thursdays were unhealthy snack night, usually nachos. Other nights, we are happy with each other and a glass of water. We also appreciate the snacks much more on those special nights.

Maybe I beat this to death, but it's super important that you get the idea: you need to establish a rigor and discipline around rewards, because the food industry and the restaurant industry are not going to do it for you. You should develop a "rhythm of rewards", again shoot for one every other day at least. Do this fairly quickly; otherwise, every available reward ends up being a yes/no spur-of-the-moment up or down decision. "Up" usually wins.

EXERCISE PREVIEW: THINK ABOUT WHAT REWARDS DO YOU PLAN FOR YOURSELF EACH WEEK. EACH MONTH?

There may be some great folks who start eating healthy and actually move away from any kind of desire for donuts or pizza. You may scoff at this, but it may be you after a few months. So don't sell it short. If you do turn out to be one of these types of people, you still get rewards. Your reward night might end up being as simple as eating salmon in a restaurant one night a week, while skipping the donuts and pizza. Not everyone is like this, so remember, its ok to have a really "bad" reward like a donut, as long as you establish a natural limit.

There are a couple of important additional hints around rewards that will help you beyond just establishing a close-ended routine.

Restaurants. Restaurants are a bane for many of us. We have the sense they are special. Maybe we were raised that they were for special occasions. So we often allow ourselves to indulge. Restaurants used to be for special occasions, but now one source estimates American's eat in or from restaurants nearly six times per week (United States Healthful Food Council, 2015). That's almost daily. For some of us, it's more than once a day. But many of us still say we can have a burger, or fries, or whatever, because we are "eating out" … every single day. If you live that life, then you can't treat it as special every time you show up.

Your food reward system should land you in a restaurant around twice per week. That should be enough to go back to the old-fashioned method of actually appreciating a restaurant meal. I know the restaurant industry is going to hate to read this, but we need to get back to the culture of making restaurants special.

This may also mean that you turn to your kitchen more frequently. This doesn't mean you have to spend more time cooking, or learning to cook in the first place. The reality is that the point of impact is the grocery store. You buy lots of fruit, vegetables, and ready-to-eat stuff at the grocery store that is reasonably healthy, then when it's time to grab a food for lunch at work, or for dinner on the go – you have a self-disciplined set of choices. Alternatively, if you say, "I'll just grab something on the way there (or home)", you end up buying yourself an un-scheduled reward. So just remember this: limit yourselves to restaurants one to three times per week.

Work. So what do I do about work? If I travel for work, I have to eat in restaurants while I'm travelling. Even when I'm in the office, the culture of the company is to break for lunch. I am a manager and I have to take an employees to lunch several times a week for motivation or morale.

If this is the case for you, it's important for you to "emasculate" those restaurant visits. Whether its lunch in the office or dinner on the road, if it's not an identified reward you need to eat like you are not in a restaurant. That means have a salad and a cup of clear soup. Otherwise many chain restaurants have healthy meals under 700 calories. Require yourself to pick one of those – like a small piece of fish, broccoli, and unsweetened ice tea. Maybe a Friday departmental lunch could be one of your weekly rewards. The rest of the days view it as a "forced visit" and stick to salad (without fried chicken, cream dressing, giant croutons, etc. as the payload).

Also, if you don't feel required to eat lunch out for work every day, I would strongly recommend that you just throw together a bag of food to take with you every day. Call this breakfast and lunch and you can eat some of it in transit. Don't include rewards generally. Throw in some carrots. A sandwich. An apple. A yogurt. Granola bars. Keep it generally healthy and shoot for 1,500 calories or so. That leaves you room for a nice dinner when you get home.

Finally, when vendors or moms leave food "for the office", just get in the habit of walking right on by. This stuff is almost never healthy and it's not an identified reward. In fact, if an employee brought it, it's usually one of those kids' un-finished food rewards that mom or dad was too horrified to feed to their own children.

Grocery stores. Get most of your food in grocery stores or produce markets. The exception should be your one- or two weekly restaurant rewards. I realize there is lots of unhealthy and fattening stuff in grocery stores, but the idea is that if you are forced to select your food, and then assemble it either for work, or for an at-home dinner, you usually will end up with a more sensible result. After all, most of us lack a pre-heated deep fryer to make perfect fries with every meal, nor do we have the patience to cook sizzling bacon to top off every chicken or beef burger.

The reality is that grocery shopping forces you to think about your food choices and consider the assembly of your food. As you think, make manageable choices. If you aren't sure what to buy, go back and re-read the chapter on nutrition. There is no quota to how much of your food you can buy in the produce section. Stay away from the store bakery. It is that easy.

I spent a lot of ink on this topic because it's so important. In society, situational rewards are constant and ubiquitous. Learn to ration your food rewards yourself. No one else will do it for you. Define 3 or 4 every week. Identify what you like and establish a pattern and fixed limit. This will keep you from blowing up, and it will also drive you to appreciate the rewards **100x more** than you do when rewards are constant. In Summary: Limit unconstrained restaurant visits to one or two per week; If you have to eat in restaurants for work, emasculate those visits by eating healthy salads or clear soup; Buy most of your food in grocery stores, not restaurants; Pick a lot of that food out of produce.

WEIGHING YOURSELF

Weighing yourself frequently is critically important for most people. You need to weigh yourself daily, and ideally twice a day. Keep an accurate scale in your bathroom. In so doing, you are turning yourself into a mini "biofeedback" device. Your brain processes what you've eaten this morning or during the past couple of days, and you start to develop an intuitive sense of relationship between cause and effect.

Some people will criticize this recommendation and say that it is obsessive. Others will remind you that your weight can vary by a few pounds over the course of the day, so that it can be misleading. It may vary because you just chugged a huge glass of water. Or if you are starting a fast, you may lose a few pounds of water weight that is not "real" weight loss. You weigh less in the morning because you are dehydrated. All this is true but distracting. The reality as that knowing the peculiarities of your weight is part of learning a rhythm of losing weight, and you will quickly train yourself to interpret the results.

I recommend you weigh yourself in the morning and at night around the same time each day so that you have consistent points of comparison. If you normally weigh 128 lbs. at night and you have three evenings in a row weighing 131 lbs., you are gaining a couple of pounds. It's important to have this feedback, because as I discussed in earlier chapters, it's hard to know precisely how many calories you've eaten on a given day, and even if you do know, it's even harder to know precisely how many you are burning.

Using the scale gives you manifest evidence on whether you have dialed down your food, and dialed up your hunger enough to achieve success. It is a tool that you use to measure and adjust until you can verify that you are in the right trajectory and have achieved the right rhythm.

RHYTHM

And so that brings us to rhythm. What is the rhythm of your weight loss? As you proceed, you will develop and refine a system and routine that enable you to consistently lose weight. You'll know when you have to dial it up, and when you are making steady consistent progress. After you reach your ideal weight, the same sense of rhythm will help you maintain it.

At first, when you begin to seek to lose weight, you may have some initial frustration or surprise that you aren't losing weight quickly. Your body is stubborn at first.   If you ever watch the show *The Biggest Loser*, you will notice that many contestants are surprised, because they think they've restricted food somewhat and are exercising, but they haven't lost any weight.   Remember that exercise doesn't use a lot of calories unless it is very intense and very long.   Reducing food is perceptual: when you start, you may think you are having smaller meals, and then your body has nagged you to eat more snacks.   As you familiarize yourself with the sensations of hunger and fasting, you'll get better and more comfortable with consuming calories in the range that will drive weight loss.

Typically, after 2 or 3 weeks of focused effort, you will begin to see consistently lower readings on the scale.   You are seeking consistent steady weight loss of 1 to 2 pounds per week.   Once you have a sense of the right routine, your weight loss will remain consistent, and you will learn to anticipate it.

You must pick a day to fast.   When you fast, you reduce your overall calories by 1/7 = 14%.   Suppose you burn 2,500 calories per day. If you fast one day, you can aim to eat with a deficit of just 500 calories on just two other days, and you'll lose about a pound per week, even if you don't create a deficit on other days.   This is actually a pretty good pattern.   Having days that you eat in rough balance gets you in practice for the rhythm you'll maintain when you reach your ideal weight.   If you pick Fridays to fast, you might also focus on reduced calories on Monday and Wednesday. Sprinkle manageable rewards on other days. Or you may decide to look at every day as a low-calorie day with the exceptions being rewards you've defined. This is a rhythm you'll find.   When it comes time to maintain your weight, or increase it if you are adding muscle, you'll find the adjustments you need to make in consumption are relatively minor.

You might find your rhythm is a steady rhythm.   I had an associate who lost over 150 pounds.   He would pick up three Subway subs every day – a six inch veggie for breakfast, a twelve inch veggie for lunch, and a twelve inch turkey for dinner.   That was his food for the day. (No his name is not Jared. This was a real acquaintance before Jared hit the scene.) He would hit the treadmill for one hour six days and fast one day per week.   He liked the certainty of having his food precisely laid out every day without having to think about it.   Although he did break my guideline of staying out of restaurants, he established a rhythm that was structured and worked for him.   Weekends would include a trip to a "real" restaurant.

Rhythm is a key element of success not addressed in a fascinating *New York Times* article about contestants of – you guessed it – *The Biggest Loser* (Kolata, 2016). The dirty secret of the legacy of "*Loser*" is that even though most contestants lose very substantial amounts of weight during the contest, the majority gain it back. In a six-year study of *Season 8* participants, 13 of 14 contestants had gained substantial weight back and 4 weighed more than they did before the contest started.

The article cites lower resting metabolism as a potential contributor: after the show contestants developed RMR about 500 calories lower than what is expected for persons their size according to the study. It is also mentioned that contestants might have lower levels of leptin, the hunger suppressing hormone. What is not directly addressed is that these contestants lived in extraordinary circumstances for *30 weeks* --- on a fitness ranch where diet and exercise are obsessively controlled by professionals. Lifestyle is comprehensively different in returning to "ordinary" lives. In particular activity and exercise can have significant impact on resting metabolic rates. Treating obesity like a metabolic disease belies the need to both exercise and develop a rhythm and routine in real life that creates a *sustainable* calorie balance. Once again, *you* have to figure out what works for you, and unnatural circumstances are never sustainable.

Here is what will happen as you establish your rhythm. It could take a couple weeks before you start consistently shedding pounds; however, if you have been doing zero exercise, just adding that hour on the treadmill will move your metabolism into a different gear, and it may start happening more quickly. If you are not shedding pounds, you need to put more stress on hunger – get comfortable with it, pick days to increase intervals between meals, and resolve to spend more time in a state of caloric restriction. Go back and re-read Chapter 4 again for inspiration. Make sure you take a full 24-hour fast every week. These are the levers you turn and the patterns you create: hunger, exercise, fasting, frequent weigh-ins (**Figure 6**).

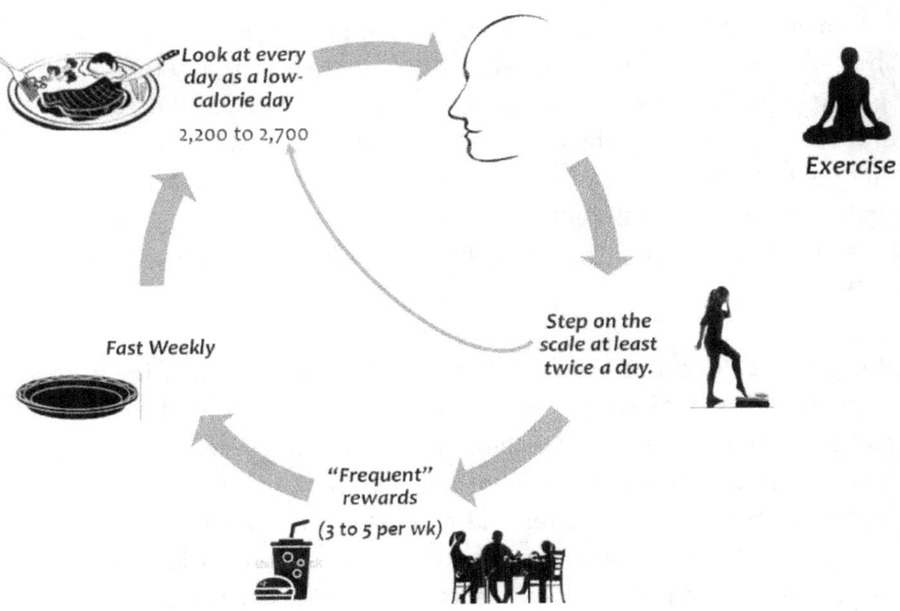

Figure 6 – Developing a rhythm for shedding weight.

Your rhythm is your rhythm. Remember that learning to be comfortable feeling hungry is one of the most important elements of an established rhythm that will help you develop control. When you have a routine – a cycle of restraint and reward, and a routine of activities that works for you, and a system that enables you to reach ideal weight, it's something you'll want to share with others struggling with weight. Doing so will motivate and inspire others. But remember your rhythm is yours. It's personal. It's exactly what works for you, but not exactly what works for everyone.

Remember the key elements of success from **Figure 6**: hunger, fasting, exercise, and rewards. Beyond this there can be a great variety of formats that will bring you to success. That is why this book has not endeavored to tell you exactly what to eat and exactly how to exercise. Hundreds of books do that, and none of them will help you. Routines that are complex to follow will not fit your lifestyle or your routines, will be challenging for you to adopt, and will mean that you quickly fall off a program.

National Weight Control Registry. To put a finer point on this topic of rhythm and self-discovery, I want to refer to the *National Weight Control Registry*. The National Weight Control Registry was founded in 1994 out of Brown University. It is believed to be the largest ongoing investigation of successful weight loss maintenance. The registry is tracking over 10,000 individuals and constantly recruiting new subjects. This trove of data has resulted in at least 30 research articles published in various peer-reviewed scientific journals tracking the progress of subjects who have lost large amounts of weight and maintained that weight loss for a long period of time. There is a lot of discussion of what works and what does not work – but yet here is a real-world trove of data of people who have been successful long term. Many of the research studies revolve around 1,000 subjects who all lost at least 30 pounds, with an average loss of 65 pounds, and maintained that loss for a minimum of 5 years. Here are some of the key findings that are consistent through numerous studies of this population (Klem, Wing, McGuire, Seagle, & Hill, 1997), (McGuire, RR, ML, & JO, 1999), (Hill, Wyatt, Phelan, & Wing, 2005).

- **Weight Loss Programs** – Slightly over half of successful participants lost weight using some kind of weight lost program, and slightly under half succeeded completely on their own. Shocking that around half used no assistive aids. This fact echoes one of the major themes in this book: if Weight Watchers or Slim Fast cures the tedium, inspires and motivates you, gets you through your day, you should buy it; but, ultimately you have to reach your ideal weight on your own, with the arrows in your mental and emotional quiver. You're no more likely to succeed with it than without it. *You* have to find your weekly rhythm of hunger and rewards that enables you to shed pounds and then maintain a target weight. *You* have to become comfortable with hunger. Our aim with this book was to inspire and motivate you, and put those arrows in your quiver. You can see from the statistics in the registry that many people used diet aids or programs, but they were not used by half of people. If you decide to use them, remember they are not a crutch. Only your own self-discovered rhythm for action and progress will lead you to success.

- **Exercise** – A whopping 94% of the successful group said they increased their physical activity or exercise. Most of the successful group was burning 1,000 to 2,000 calories per week in the gym, consistent with the 3 to 5 hour weekly recommendation I have made in this book. The most frequently reported type of exercise was **walking** the same modality I recommend for you if you are obese and just beginning to lose weight. *At least three separate studies* in the *Weight Control Registry* database noted the high level of regular exercise among persons who lost significant weight, even though, as I have discussed the total calories burned in exercise may not be highly significant.

- **Weighing Yourself** – Successful people weigh themselves to monitor progress and maintenance. It turns out that **75% of the successful subjects weighed themselves** at least weekly. Remember this is with the average subject in the registry having kept off 65 pounds for over 5 years. Seventy five percent of these subjects are still weighing themselves! Further, 45% are weighing themselves either daily or more than once per day. *At least three separate studies* in the weight control registry observed very high levels of self-weighing among those who were successful at losing significant weight and maintain it for a long period of time.

- **Maintenance of Lost Weight** – this is one of the most fascinating findings in the weight loss registry and one that seems to contradict conventional wisdom: most subjects reported that once they reached a target weight, keeping the weight off was easy. Sixty-eight percent of successful subjects rated maintenance of target weight as either "easy" or "moderately easy" (Klem, Wing, McGuire, Seagle, & Hill, 1997). You may recall some of these themes in this book: once you find your rhythm for shedding weight, and balance hunger and reward, you'll begin to lose weight. If you've been maintaining your weight at 300 pounds with no further weight gain, you may be again eating similar calories when you reach 150 pounds. Maintaining ideal weight can involve eating slightly more calories than when losing weight. If you understand your rhythms for eating and losing, if you weigh yourself frequently, it's easy to be successful in maintenance. We have the perception that maintaining lost weight is difficult because so many people who seek to lose a few pounds do it with a frenzy of ad hoc food restrictions that are not sustainable, and never learn a rhythm of eating, exercise, and rewards that they can use permanently. Most due lose some pounds, but never reach their ideal weight even for a day.

- **Health and Happiness** – Nearly all successful registry members indicated that weight loss led to improvements in their level of **energy, physical mobility, general mood, self-confidence,** and **physical health** – over 90% reported results in every one of these categories. Also not a new discussion for us, going all the way back to Chapter 1. The combination of reaching your ideal weight and engaging in exercise will make you feel younger, more energetic, and more optimistic. Everyone tends to believe the manifest medical benefits of correct weight (lower incidence of diabetes, heart disease, etc.), but there is less understanding of energy and well-being. Not only will the likelihood of long term health problems like diabetes, heart disease, and cancer be greatly diminished, but you will do more and you will be more productive.

What you should have concluded in considering all this is that successful people have learned the things that matter in moving you to reach your ideal weight. They understand what works and they act in their own interests. You can be successful if you empower yourself to model proven successful behaviors.

SUMMARY AND CONCLUSIONS

We've covered a lot of ground in eight chapters. Hopefully this is a starting point for you. Hopefully you are motivated and fired up. If you decide to reach your ideal weight, in a few weeks you'll be moving at a steady pace toward that goal. In Chapter 1, I hope I motivated you to reach your ideal weight by reminding you that you will live a life of poor health and rapid aging if you decide to live fat. You'll be less successful and productive, you'll have lower self-esteem, and you'll have poorer relationships and interactions with those who surround you.

In Chapter 2 and Chapter 3, I taught you how to calculate your ideal weight and how much you can eat to reach and maintain it. Most people need about 2,200 to 2,500 calories per week to maintain their weight. If you create a deficit of around 500 calories per day from this level, you will lose about a pound a week. Use Chapters 2 and 3 as mini-companions to enable you to establish the goals for weight and eating that you need for success.

In Chapter 4, I talked about hunger. Hunger is important. It is your main weapon to lose weight. Most programs that aim to help you lose weight aim to help you deal with hunger. Hunger is natural and part of the metabolic cycle. Constant satiety is an artifact of the modern society. We are all addicted to food, but people are different in how they handle hunger. You need to learn to become comfortable with hunger yourself. Many diet programs don't work, because they promise you that you can lose weight without feeling hungry. Even massive interventions like gastric bypass surgery are focused on handling hunger. There is significant evidence that these surgeries are not a permanent solution for many people. If this is true, the reason for failure is that the surgery does not permanently eliminate the essential requirement that persons need to learn to address hunger. Hunger should be your beacon that your body is entering those essential metabolic states where fat is used as fuel. You should learn to embrace that.

In Chapter 5, I discussed Fasting. Fasting is essential for successful weight loss and you should enjoy one 24-hour fast every week. Fasting drives your body into the metabolic state of ketosis (fat burning). It's hard to train your body to burn fat by creating a tiny calorie deficit every day. Your body usually nags you with hunger to get you to eat a bit more and usually wins. Fasting teaches you to be comfortable with hunger and allows you to create a substantial calorie deficit over the course of every week. Fasting drives autophagy (cellular clean-up) and many studies in animals and people have shown it contributes to energy, mental acuity, well-being, and longevity.

In Chapter 6 I talked about nutrition. Nutrition is somewhat of a sideshow when it comes to reaching your ideal weight. In substance, how much you eat and your level of activity determine your weight, and what you eat is not as important. It may be important for other aspects of health, but not weight. Among the three main categories of macronutrients, there are no pure villains. Carbs are the closest thing: Your body doesn't need them for structure or functioning, only for fuel. They are very dense sources of fuel so it is easy to eat way too much when you include carbohydrates. Push them aside, use whole grains which deliver energy slowly, or treat them as a small-portion treat. Fats are healthy and essential and they don't make you fat. Most scientists think unsaturated fats are the healthiest (fish, canola, nut oils) and you should eat these without guilt. Some scientists think saturated fats contribute to heart disease (milk, cheese, beef and fatty animal protein). They may do this by increasing your cholesterol. Your liver makes the cholesterol in your blood stream, and it isn't certain that saturated fats cause it to be elevated beyond the impact of eating too much food overall. Have your cholesterol checked by a doctor. If it's in a healthy range after you reach your ideal weight, you don't need to worry about avoiding saturated fats. Finally, eat all the fruits and vegetables you want. These take up a lot of room, have low calorie density, and contain the micronutrients your body needs. It's nearly impossible to overeat with vegetables.

In Chapter 7, I discussed exercise. You don't have to exercise a lot. As little as 25 minutes a day can be enough. It will fit any lifestyle. The extra energy you feel and the lack of low-productivity afternoon dips will more than make up for the invested time. Make sure you reach high intensity every time you exercise. Get your heart rate to 80% of your logical max and hold it there for several minutes. You should engage in structured exercise 5 times a week. Four times is ok. You need to be selfish about exercise rather than finding excuses not to do it. The calories burned in exercise are fairly small – maybe 250 calories in an hour of light walking or jogging – but exercise gives you the energy, focus, and optimism that you need for success. Several studies of participants in the *National Weight Control Registry*, which tracks persons who have lost substantial weight and kept it off for a long time have concluded that over 90% of successful persons exercise 4 or 5 times per week.

In Chapter 8 I talked about putting everything together. After you calculate your ideal weight and get a sense how much you can eat every day to lose a pound per week, you have all the arrows you need in your quiver to get you to your goal: using hunger and frequent weighings as beacons. Hunger tells you that you are losing weight. Engaging in a weekly fast. Engaging in exercise 4 or 5 times per week. Weighing yourself very frequently. Getting comfortable with hunger. If you don't see weight coming off after a of couple weeks, get a little more comfortable with hunger: pick low calorie days to blend in with your weekly fast. Make sure you plan frequent reasonable rewards to keep yourself motivated. You will discover your own rhythm for weight loss and once you have understand that rhythm, you'll consistently lose weight. Once you are at your ideal weight, you can eat on average 500 calories more per day to maintain it. Not a wholesale life changer, but you've learned a routine and you know how to reward yourself. Successful persons in the *National Weight Control Registry* generally report that maintenance is not that difficult, despite conventional wisdom.

YOUR PLACE IN THE UNIVERSE

You are meant to live a long, happy life. You should deserve it. It is very difficult to do that if you are overweight. If you are just 20- or 25 pounds overweight, you may not even realize the impact it is having on your sense of health, well-being, and energy. If you are 70 pounds overweight, you have a deadly disease. As you age that disease will fell you with one of the most common killers of men and women: diabetes, heart disease, cancer.

Many products and diets try to tell you that you can lose weight by not feeling hungry. Food is something everyone is addicted to. A feeling of hunger is natural. You can discover your own rhythms of hunger, eating, and rewards that enable you to reach and maintain your ideal weight. You will find and discover that certain foods, certain patterns of eating, certain patterns of fasting, and certain patterns of thought increase satiety, and enable you to become comfortable with hunger.

Today you are assaulted by many claims of food simplicity – organic, non-GMO, all natural, gluten free, free range – that aim to make you feel you are eating healthy. In reality, the greatest threat to your health and longevity is eating too much food. These other claims might have an infinitesimal impact on nebulous ideas of disease, but there is, as of yet, no proof. Additionally, these products are often not very green – using more land and resources to be produced than alternatives. Deforestation and habitat destruction is one of the greatest environmental threats faced by growing populations and civilizations (Diamond, 2005). If you want to eat healthy food, eat fruits and vegetables immoderately and don't be distracted by spurious health claims.

In the same vein, the amount of unnecessary food you are consuming in order to maintain your excess weight has an impact on all the world around you. How many eggs do you eat per day for breakfast … in baked goods … recipes? A chicken makes one egg per day. A farmer has to keep one chicken, alive, fed, cleaned, and composted for every daily egg you eat. If you eat meat, consider how many cows you eat each year with the steaks, hamburgers, and taco meat. Each cow needs 2 acres of pasture to sustain it. How many acres are out are maintaining your habit? Then add pigs, fish, lambs, and other animals. Next consider the salad you had for dinner last night … how many acres and water did that use? Consider further all the trips to the bathroom, to poop out that food. The extra toilet flushes, and the need to treat that extra sewage. Consider the extra cotton grown to make large clothes, and the extra fuel burned to carry a heavy person from New York to Los Angeles on a plane. I'm not trying to burden you guilt, but rather to make the point of considering that we should view food as a gracious gift, never to be wasted, always to be enjoyed, and to be consumed in the minimum practical necessary amount.

Enough guilt. This book was written to inspire and motivate you to reach your ideal weight. Now you have a sound framework to tackle that challenge, and I hope now the motivation and dedication to be permanently successful.

Exercises – Chapter 8 *Holism*

Last writing exercise. These questions will help you think about a rhythm that can help you maintain your ideal weight.

1. **When do you feel the most stressed every week? What could you do about it?**

Stressor	What I Could Do About It
1.	
2.	

2. **When could you reserve time for exercise four or five days a week? Your solution needs to be consistent, repeatable, not pre-emptible, and not general ("while kids are doing homework = no good")**

When	How

3. What are good times or occasions to reward yourself every week?

When	How

4. What factors or mileposts drive rhythm and consistency in your week? Work, Friday night, Sunday football? List the key rhythmic events on your week. Frequent weighing helps you to predict and maintain your weight as you pass through the rhythm of your week.

When	What

Believe in consistency. Believe in your ability to succeed!

Amandine Chaix, A. Z. (2014, December 2). Time-Restricted Feeding Is a Preventative and Therapeutic Intervention against Diverse Nutritional Challenges. *Cell Metabolism, 20*(6), 991-1005.

Bock, L. (2015). *Work Rules.* New York: Twelve Hachette Book Group.

C He, M. B.-D. (2012, Jan 18). Exercise-induced BCL2-regulated autophagy is required for muscle glucose homeostasis. *481*(7382), 511-515.

Campbell, J. V. (2015, April 7). *8 Fatty Foods with Health Benefits*. Retrieved from Mens Health: http://www.menshealth.com/nutrition/fatty-foods-health-benefits

Celiac Disease Foundation. (2015). *Celiac Disease*. Retrieved from Celiac Disease Foundation: celiac.org

Consumer Reports. (2015, September). p. 15.

Dalton Conley, R. G. (2015). Gender, Body Mass and Economic Status. *The National Bureau of Economic Research*, 1 and ff.

David Zinczenko, P. M. (2013). *The 8-Hour Diet: Watch the Pounds Disappear without Watching What You Eat!* New York: Rodale Books.

Devlin, K. (2009). *Top 10 Reasons Why The BMI Is Bogus.* Washington, DC: National Public Radio.

Diamond, J. (2005). *Collapse: How Societies Choose to Fail or Succeed.* New York: Penguin Group.

Gifford, B. (2015). *Spring Chicken - Stay Young Forever (Or Die Trying).* New York: Grand Central Publishing.

Hill, J., Wyatt, H., Phelan, S., & Wing, R. (2005, Jul-Aug). The National Weight Control Registry: is it useful in helping deal with our obesity epidemic. *Journal of Nutritional Education and Behavior, 37*(4), 206-10.

KA Gudzune, R. D. (2015, April 7). Efficacy of commercial weight-loss programs: an updated systematic review. *Annals of Internal Medicine, 162*(7), 501-512.

Katz., D. (2015, October 26). *Is All Saturated Fat the Same?* Retrieved from Huffpost Healthy Living: http://www.huffingtonpost.com/david-katz-md/saturated-fat_b_875401.html

KD Tipton, R. W. (2001, March). Exercise, protein metabolism, and muscle growth. *Int J Sport Nutr Exerc Metab, 11*(1), 109-132.

Kevin D Hall, e. a. (2011). Quantification of the Effect of Energy Imbalance on Body Weight. *The Lancet, 378*, 826-837.

Klem, M., Wing, R., McGuire, M., Seagle, H., & Hill, J. (1997, Aug). A descriptive study of individuals successful at long-term maintenance of substantial weight loss. *American Journal of Clinical Nutrition, 66*(2), 239-46.

Kolata, G. (2016, May 2). After 'The Biggest Loser' Their Bodies Fought to Regain Weight. *The New York Times*.

Lazarus, S. (2012, February 6). *A Hundred Years Ago*. Retrieved from ahundredyearsago.com: http://ahundredyearsago.com/2012/02/06/average-height-for-males-and-females-in-1912-and-2012/

Loftus, P. (2015, March 17). Weight-Loss Drugs Face Hesitant Patients. *The Wall Street Journal*, p. D1.

M Alirezaei, C. K. (2010, August). Short-term fasting induces profound neuronal autophagy. *Autophagy, 6*(6), 702-710.

Marie Dunford, J. A. (2015). *Nutrition for Sports and Exercise* (3rd ed.). Stamford, CT: Cenage Learning.

Mark D Mifflin, S. T. (1990, February). A new predictive equation for resting energy expenditure in healthy individuals. *The American Journal of Clinical Nutrition, 51*(2), 241-247.

Martin B, M. M. (2006). Caloric restriction and intermittent fasting: Two potential diets for successful brain aging. *Ageing Res Rev., 5*(3), 332-353.

Mattson MP, W. R. (2005, March). Beneficial effects of intermittent fasting and caloric restriction on the cardiovascular and cerebrovascular systems. *J Nutr Biochem, 16*(3), 129-137.

McGinty, J. C. (2015, January 9). Fit for Motivation, if Not Precision. *The Wall Street Journal*.

McGinty, J. C. (2015, August 28). The Difficulty in Taking a Bite out of Food Waste. *The Wall Street Journal*.

McGuire, M., RR, W., ML, K., & JO, H. (1999, Jul). Behavioral strategies of individuals who have maintained long-term weight losses. *Obesity Research, 7*(4), 334-41.

Murphy, J. (2015, July 7). PGA's Padraig Harrington Gets Back Into the Golf Swing. *The Wall Street Journal*, p. D3.

Natashalh. (2014, June 30). *Were People Shorter in the Past? Average Height 'Back Then'*. Retrieved from HubPages: http://hubpages.com/hub/Myths-and-misconceptions-about-history-people-were-shorter-back-then

Peart, K. N. (2015, February 16). Anti-inflammatory mechanism of dieting and fasting revealed. *Yale News*, p. 2015.

Puzziferri, e. a. (2014, September 3). Long-term Follow-up After Bariatric Surgery - A Systematic Review. *The Journal of the American Medical Association, 312*(9), 934-942.

Robert H. Lustig, K. M.-C.-M. (2015, October 26). Isocaloric fructose restriction and metabolic improvement in children with obesity and metabolic syndrome. *Obesity*. doi:10.1002/oby.21371

Sahu, A. (2003). Leptin signaling in the hypothalamus: emphasis on energy homeostasis and leptin resistance. *Frontiers in Neuroendocrinology, 24*(4), 225-253.

Singer-Vine, J. (2009, July 20). *Beyond BMI - Why doctors won't stop using an outdated measure for obesity*. Retrieved from Slate: http://www.slate.com/articles/health_and_science/science/2009/07/beyond_b mi.2.html

Siri-Tarino PW, S. Q. (2010). Meta-analysis of prospective cohort studies evaluating the association of saturated fat with cardiovascular disease. *American Journal of Clinical Nutrition, 91*(3), 535-546.

Tergesen, A. (2014, December 1). Why Everything You Know About Aging is Probably Wrong. *The Wall Street Journal*, pp. R1-R2.

United States Healthful Food Council. (2015). *About*. Retrieved from United States Healthful Food Council: ushfc.org/about

Valter D. Longo, C. E. (2003, February 28). Evolutionary Medicine: From Dwarf Model Systems to Healthy Centenarians? *Science, 299*(5611), 1342-1346.

Varady, K. (2013). *The Every-Other-Day Diet: The Diet That Lets You Eat All You Want (Half the Time) and Keep the Weight Off*. New York: Hyperion.

W Willet, A. A. (1994, May). Trans Fatty Acids: Are the Effects Only Marginal? *American Journal of Public Health, 84*(5), 722-724.

Wade, N. (2011, February 16). Ecuadorean Villagers May Hold Secret to Longevity. *The New York Times*, p. A6.

Wang, S. S. (2015, June 29). Science Wants to Know: Can Worms Swim? *The Wall Street Journal*, p. D5.

Yun-Hee Youm, K. Y. (2015). The ketone metabolite β-hydroxybutyrate blocks NLRP3 inflammasome–mediated inflammatory disease. *Nature Medicine, 21*, 263-269. doi:10.1038/nm.3804

List of Figures

List of Tables

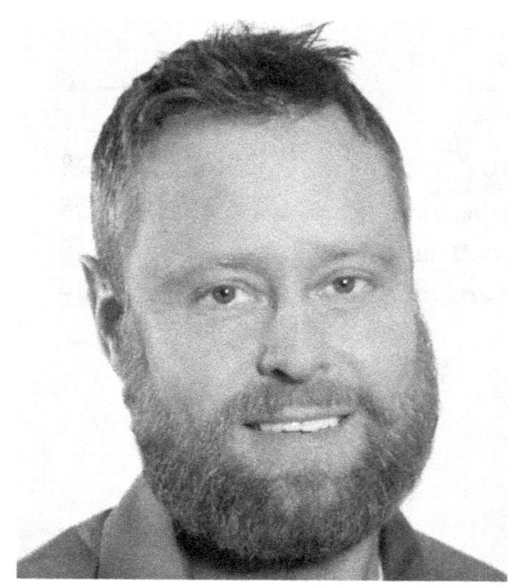

Mike Woosley earned his Ph.D. in engineering from The University of Virginia and has done stints working at Los Alamos National Lab, Oak Ridge National Lab, and for the Atomic Energy Commission in France.

Since 1999 Mike, has worked as an officer at a string of companies in digital media, usually related to the technology and optimization that make media and information free, fast, and ubiquitous.

Mike starting thinking about *Ideal Weight* when he realized that many lethargic adults attribute lack of energy to aging, when it's actually related to weight. He noticed that many adults less than 30 pounds overweight don't realize they are overweight, or that excess weight is sapping energy and optimism. Mike started experimenting with intermittent fasting in 2006, and has been amazed and elated by the string of compelling research and public awareness of the necessity and benefits of this technique in improving health.

Mike is an NSPA certified personal trainer. In his spare time, Mike enjoys playing hockey, cooking, eating, solving brain-bending puzzles, landscaping, and fixing everything that four kids break around the house.

Instagram: mikewoosley
Twitter: @DrWoosley

Acknowledgment

Thank you to Sherri for her patience, encouragement and tolerance. Thank you to all my beta readers for their great feedback.